The Simply Renal Diet Cookbook

Low Sodium, Potassium, and Phosphorus Easy and Healthy Renal Diet Recipes to Help You Manage Kidney Disease

Beryl Ramirez

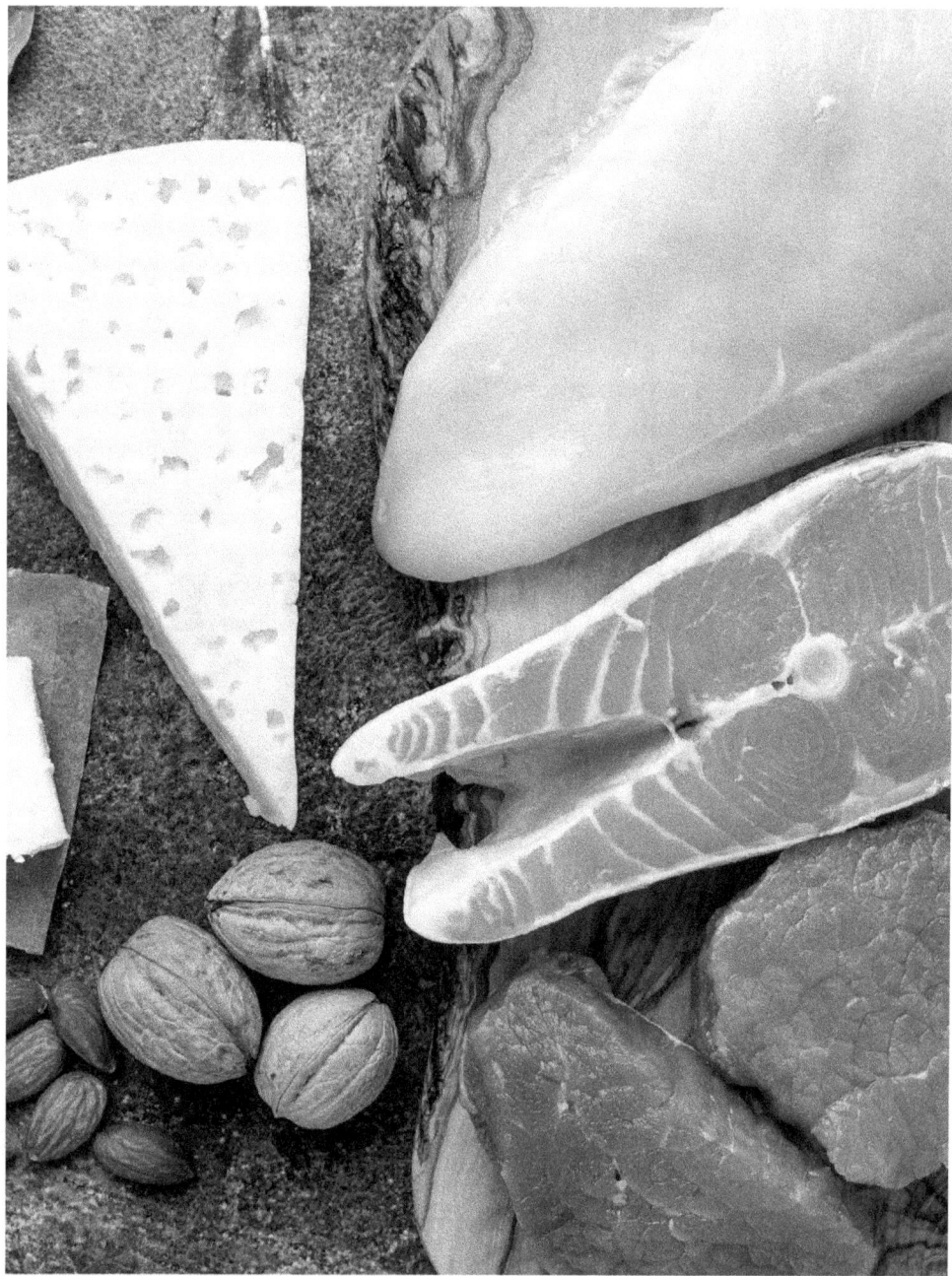

Table of Content

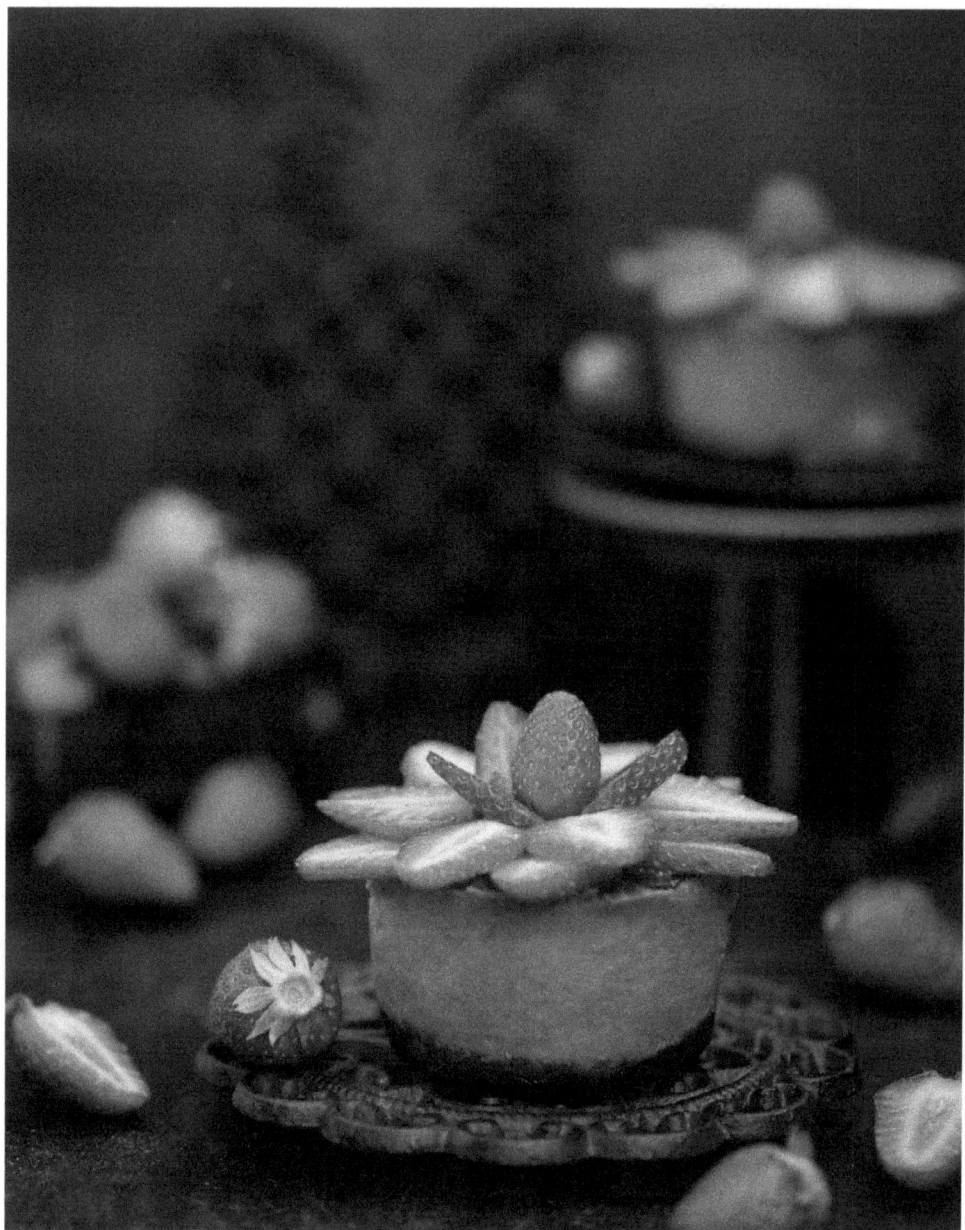

INTRODUCTION

Changing your diet is not as limiting as you think: many whole foods can easily replace refined, processed foods all too common in everyday meals. Many simple snacks and easy foods to eat on the go can fit well into a renal diet. It's a culinary journey that can boost your body's vital functions, in addition to improving your kidneys by reducing the amount of waste produced. Diet is one of the most important factors in our health. What we eat today determines how well we live and function tomorrow. When we have a choice at a better life, despite the challenges of renal failure, it's crucial to take action as soon as possible to ensure we have the best opportunity to live life to the fullest and make the most of our choices.

The renal diet focuses primarily on supporting kidney health but in doing so, you'll improve many other aspects of your health, as well. It can also be customized to fit all levels of kidney disease, from early stages and minor infections to more significant renal impairment and dialysis. Preventing the later stages is the main goal, though reaching this stage can still be treated with careful consideration of your dietary choices. In addition to medical treatment, the diet provides a way for you to gain control over your health and progression. It can mean the difference between a complete renal failure or a manageable chronic condition, where you can lead a regular, enjoyable life despite having kidney issues.

Whether or not the medication is a part of your treatment plan, your diet takes on a significant role in the health of your kidneys. Some herbs and vitamins can boost the medicinal properties found in foods and give your kidneys additional support, while limiting other ingredients which, in excess, can lead to complete renal failure if there are already signs of kidney impairment.

Thanks to this cookbook you will discover numerous recipes that will help you take care of your kidneys and have a healthy lifestyle

Food to Eat

The renal diet aims to cut down the amount of waste in the blood. When people have kidney dysfunction, the kidneys are unable to remove and filter waste properly. When waste is left in the blood, it can affect the electrolyte levels of the patient. With a kidney diet, kidney function is promoted, and the progression of complete kidney failure is slowed down.

The renal diet follows a low intake of protein, phosphorus, and sodium. It is necessary to consume high-quality protein and limit some fluids. For some people, it is important to limit calcium and potassium.

In a renal diet, here are the substances which are critical to be monitored:

Sodium and its role in the body

 Most natural foods contain sodium. Some people think that sodium and salt are interchangeable. However, salt is a compound of chloride and sodium. There might be either salt or sodium in other forms in the food we eat. Due to the added salt, processed foods include a higher level of sodium.

Apart from potassium and chloride, sodium is one of the most crucial electrolyte for the body. The main function of electrolytes is controlling the fluids when they are going in and out of the body's cells and tissues.

With sodium:

- Blood volume and pressure are regulated

- Muscle contraction and nerve function are regulated

- The acid-base balance of the blood is regulated

- The amount of fluid the body eliminates and keeps is balanced

Why is it important to monitor sodium intake for people with kidney issues?

Since the kidneys of kidney disease patients are unable to reduce excess fluid and sodium from the body adequately, too much sodium might be harmful. As fluid and sodium build up in the bloodstream and tissues, they might cause:

- Edema: swelling in face, hands, and legs

- Increased thirst

- High blood pressure

- Shortness of breath

- Heart failure

The ways to monitor sodium intake:

- Avoid processed foods

- Be attentive to serving sizes

- Read food labels

- Utilize fresh meats instead of processed

- Choose fresh fruits and veggies

- Compare brands, choosing the ones with the lowest sodium levels

- Utilize spices that do not include salt

- Ensure the sodium content is less than 400 mg per meal and not more than 150 mg per snack

- Cook at home, not adding salt

Foods to eat with lower sodium content:

- Fresh meats, dairy products, frozen veggies, and fruits

- Fresh herbs and seasonings like rosemary, oregano, dill, lime, cilantro, onion, lemon, and garlic

- Corn tortilla chips, pretzels, no salt added crackers, unsalted popcorn

Potassium and its role in the body

The main function of potassium is keeping muscles working correctly and the heartbeat regular. This mineral is responsible for maintaining electrolyte and fluid balance in the bloodstream. The kidneys regulate the proper amount of potassium in the body, expelling excess amounts in the urine.

Monitoring potassium intake

- Limit high potassium food

- Select only fresh fruits and veggies

- Limit dairy products and milk to 8 oz per day

- Avoid potassium chloride

- Read labels on packaged foods

- Avoid seasonings and salt substitutes with potassium

Foods to eat with lower potassium:

Fruits: watermelon, tangerines, pineapple, plums, peaches, pears, papayas, mangoes, lemons and limes, honeydew, grapefruit/grapefruit juice, grapes/grape juice, clementine/satsuma, cranberry juice, berries, and apples/ applesauce, apple juice.

Veggies: summer squash (cooked), okra, mushrooms (fresh), lettuce, kale, green beans, eggplant, cucumber, corn, onions (raw), celery, cauliflower, carrots, cabbage, broccoli (fresh), bamboo shoots (canned), and bell peppers

Plain Turkish delights, marshmallows and jellies, boiled fruit sweets, and peppermints

Shortbread, ginger nut biscuits, plain digestives

Plain flapjacks and cereal bars

Plain sponge cakes like Madeira cake, lemon sponge, jam sponge

Corn-based and wheat crisps

Whole grain crispbreads and crackers

Protein and other foods (bread (not whole grain), pasta, noodles, rice, eggs, canned tuna, turkey (white meat), and chicken (white meat)

Phosphorus and its role in the body

This mineral is essential in bone development and maintenance. Phosphorus helps in the development of connective organs and tissue and assists in muscle movement. Excess phosphorus is be removed by healthy kidneys. However, it is impossible with kidney dysfunction. High levels of phosphorus make bones weak by pulling calcium out of them. It might lead to dangerous calcium deposits in the heart, eyes, lungs, and blood vessels.

Monitoring phosphorus intake

- Pay attention to serving size

- Eat fresh fruits and veggies

- Eat smaller portions of foods that are rich in protein

- Avoid packaged foods

- Keep a food journal

Foods to eat with low phosphorus level:

- grapes, apples

- lettuce, leeks

- Carbohydrates (white rice, corn, and rice Cereal, popcorn, pasta, crackers (not wheat), white bread)

- Meat (sausage, fresh meat)

Food to Avoid

Food with high sodium content:

Onion salt, marinades, garlic salt, teriyaki sauce, and table salt

Pepperoni, bacon, ham, lunch meat, hot dogs, sausage, processed meats

Ramen noodles, canned produce, and canned soups

Marinara sauce, gravy, salad dressings, soy sauce, BBQ sauce, and ketchup

Chex Mix, salted nuts, Cheetos, crackers, and potato chips

Fast food

Food with a high potassium level:

Fruits: dried fruit, oranges/orange juice, prunes/prune juice, kiwi, nectarines, dates, cantaloupe, bananas, black currants, damsons, cherries, grapes, and apricots.

Vegetables: tomatoes/tomato sauce/tomato juice, sweet potatoes, beans, lentils, split peas, spinach (cooked), pumpkin, potatoes, mushrooms (cooked), chile peppers, chard, Brussels sprouts (cooked), broccoli (cooked), baked beans, avocado, butternut squash, and acorn squash.

Protein and other foods: peanut butter, molasses, granola, chocolate, bran, sardines, fish, bacon, ham, nuts and seeds, yogurt, milkshakes, and milk.

Coconut-based snacks, nut-based snacks, fudge, and toffee.

Cakes containing marzipan.

Potato crisps.

Foods with high phosphorus:

<u>Dairy products:</u> pudding, ice cream, yogurt, cottage cheese, cheese, and milk.

<u>Nuts and seeds:</u> sunflower seeds, pumpkin seeds, pecans, peanut butter, pistachios, cashews, and almonds.

<u>Dried beans and peas:</u> soybeans, split peas, refried beans, pinto beans, lentils, kidney beans, garbanzo beans, black beans, and baked beans.

<u>Meat:</u> veal, turkey, liver, lamb, beef, bacon, fish, and seafood.

<u>Carbohydrates:</u> whole grain products, oatmeal, and bran cereals.

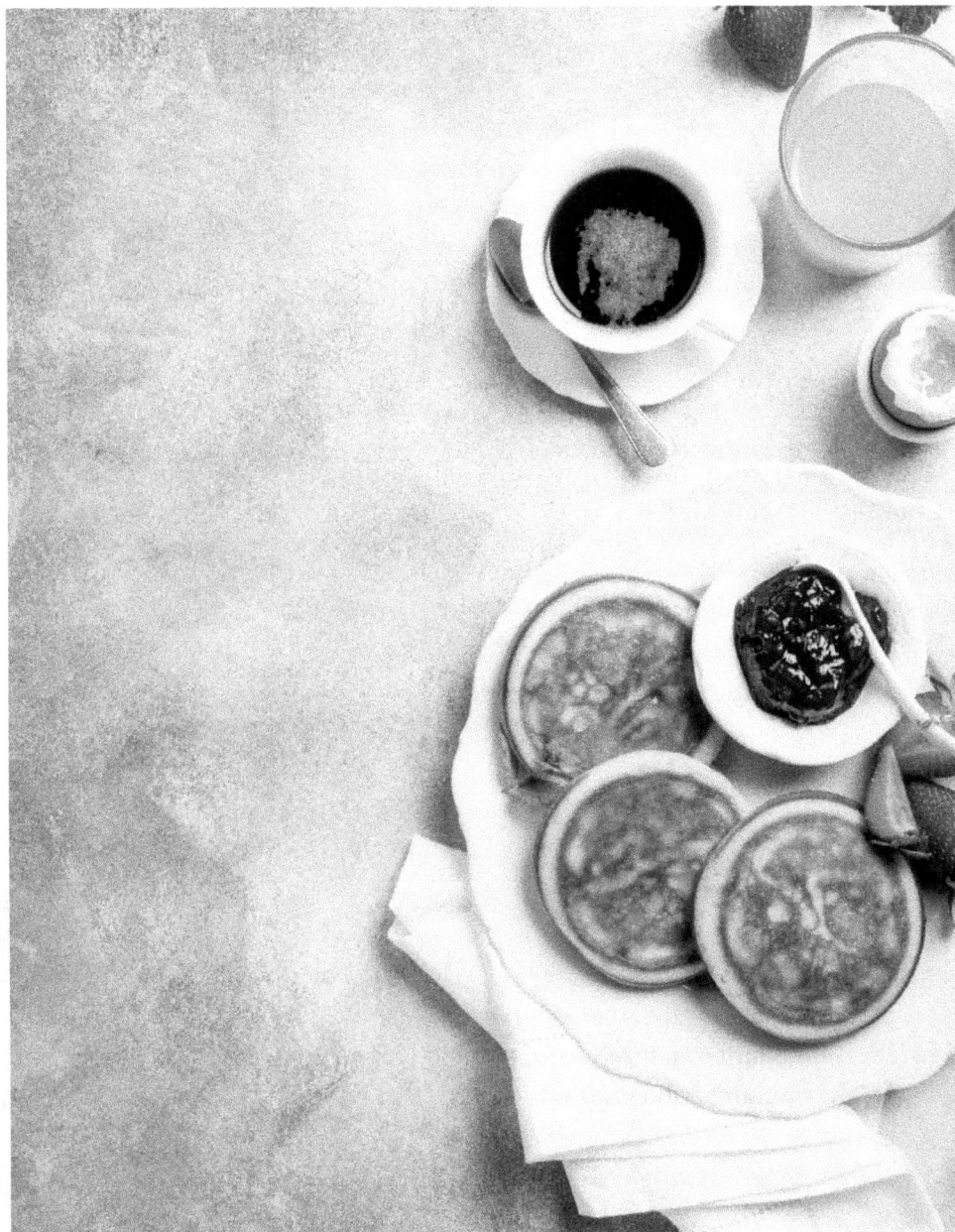

Breakfast

Simple Green Shake

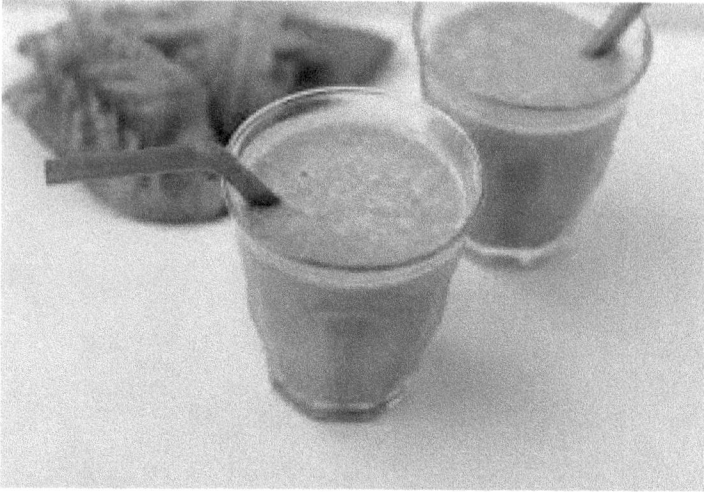

Preparation Time: 10 minutes

Cooking Time: 0 Minutes

Serving: 1

INGREDIENTS:

- ¾ cup whole milk yogurt
- 2½ cups lettuce, mix salad greens
- 1 pack stevia
- 1 tablespoon MCT oil
- 1 tablespoon chia seeds
- 1 ½ cups of water

DIRECTIONS:

1) Add listed ingredients to a blender.
2) Blend until you have a smooth and creamy texture.
3) Serve chilled and enjoy!

NUTRITION (Per Serving):

Calories: 320; Fat: 24g; Phosphorus: 30mg; Potassium: 14mg; Sodium: 11mg; Carbohydrates: 17g; Protein: 10g.

Green Beans and Roasted Onion

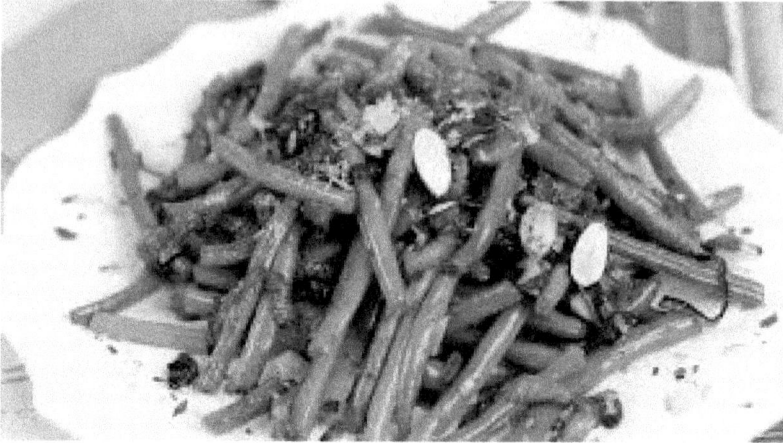

Preparation Time: 10 minutes

Cooking Time: 15 minutes

Serving: 2

INGREDIENTS:

- 1 yellow onion, sliced into rings
- ½ teaspoon onion powder
- 2 tablespoons coconut flour
- 1 1/3 pounds fresh green beans, trimmed and chopped
- ½ tablespoon salt

DIRECTIONS:

1) Take a large bowl and mix the salt with the onion powder and coconut flour.
2) Add onion rings.
3) Mix well to coat.
4) Spread the rings in the baking sheet, lined with parchment paper.
5) Drizzle with some oil.
6) Bake for 10 minutes at 400°F.

7) Parboil the green beans for 3 to 5 minutes in the boiling water.
8) Drain and serve the beans with the baked onion rings.
9) Serve warm and enjoy!

NUTRITION (Per Serving): Calories: 214; Fat: 19.4g; Phosphorus: 36mg; Potassium: 194mg; Sodium: 31mg; Carbohydrates:3.7g; Protein: 8.3g.

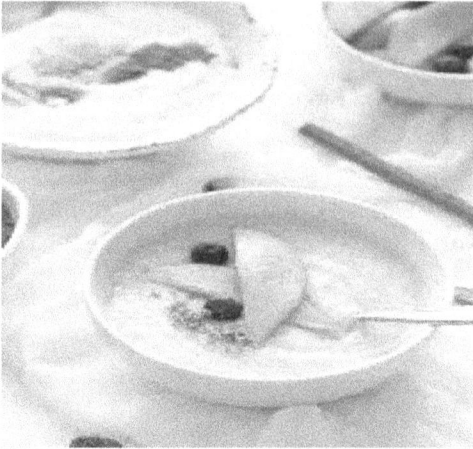

Fine Morning Porridge

Preparation Time: 15 minutes

Cooking Time: Nil

Serving: 2

INGREDIENTS:

- 2 tablespoons coconut flour
- 2 tablespoons vanilla protein powder
- 3 tablespoons Golden Flaxseed meal
- 1 ½ cups almond milk, unsweetened
- Powdered erythritol

DIRECTIONS:

1) Take a bowl and mix in flaxseed meal, protein powder, coconut flour and mix well.
2) Add mix to the saucepan (placed over medium heat).
3) Add almond milk and stir, let the mixture thicken.
4) Add your desired amount of sweetener and serve.
5) Enjoy!

NUTRITION (Per Serving): Calories: 259; Fat: 13g; Phosphorus: 30mg; Potassium: 124mg; Sodium: 31mg; Carbohydrates: 5g; Protein: 16g.

Hungarian's Porridge

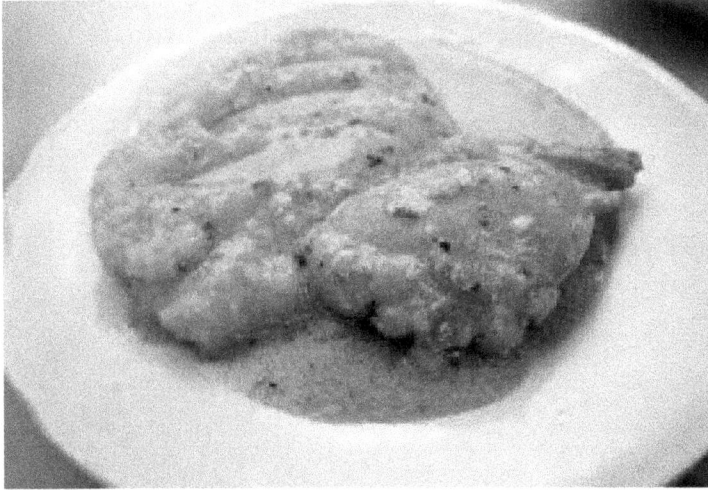

Preparation Time: 10 minutes

Cooking Time: 5-10 minutes

Serving: 2

INGREDIENTS:

- o 1 tablespoon chia seeds
- o 1 tablespoon ground flaxseed
- o 1/3 cup coconut cream
- o ½ cup of water
- o 1 teaspoon vanilla extract
- o 1 tablespoon almond butter

DIRECTIONS:

1) Add chia seeds, coconut cream, flaxseed, water, and vanilla to a small pot.
2) Stir and let it sit for 5 minutes.
3) Add butter and place pot over low heat.
4) Keep stirring as butter melts.
5) Once the porridge is hot/not boiling, pour into a bowl.

6) Add a few berries or a dash of cream for extra flavor.

NUTRITION (Per Serving): Calories: 410; Fat: 38g; Phosphorus: 30mg; Potassium: 100mg; Sodium: 11mg; Carbohydrates: 10g; Protein: 6g.

Awesome Nut Porridge

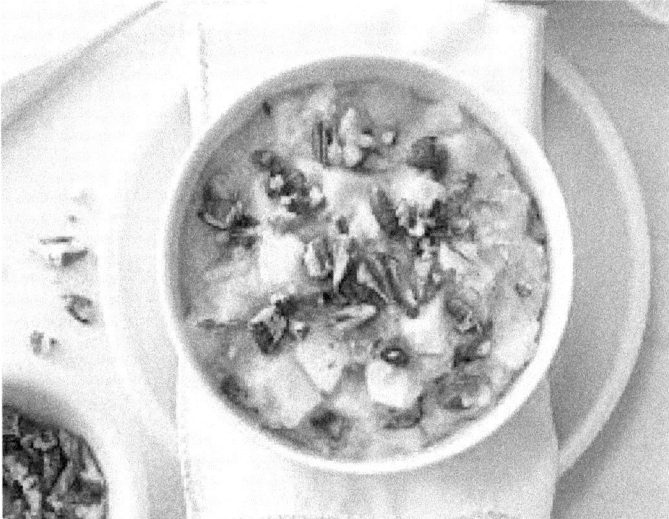

Preparation Time: 10 minutes

Cooking Time: 15 minutes

Serving: 2

INGREDIENTS:

- 1 cup cashew nuts, raw and unsalted
- 1 cup pecan, halved
- 2 tablespoons stevia
- 4 teaspoons coconut oil, melted
- 2 cups of water

DIRECTIONS:

1) Chop the nuts in a food processor and form a smooth paste.
2) Add water, oil, stevia to the nut paste and transfer the mix to a saucepan.
3) Stir cook for 5 minutes on high heat.
4) Reduce heat to low and simmer for 10 minutes.
5) Serve warm and enjoy!

NUTRITION (Per Serving): Calories: 260; Fat: 22g; Phosphorus: 15mg; Potassium: 124mg; Sodium: 30mg; Carbohydrates: 13g; Protein: 6g.

Super Scrambled Eggs

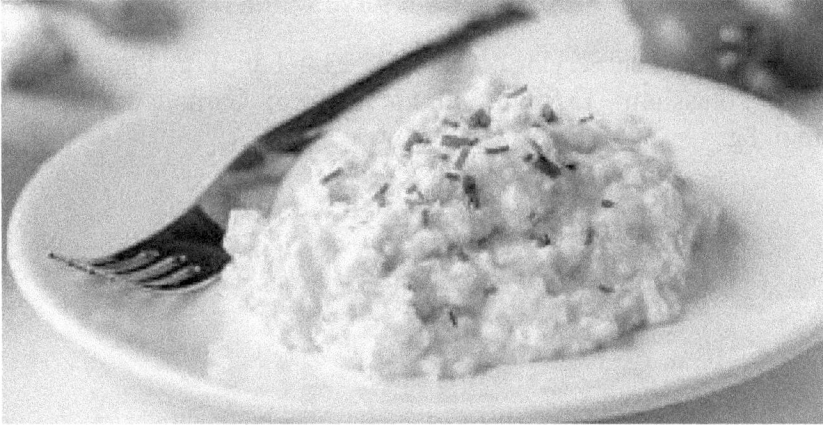

Preparation Time: 10minutes

Cooking Time: 10 minutes

Serving: 1

INGREDIENTS:

- ½ cup cream cheese
- ¼ cup unsweetened almond or rice milk
- 3 eggs
- 2 egg whites
- 1 tablespoon finely chopped scallion, green part only
- 2 tablespoons unsalted butter
- 1 tablespoon chopped fresh tarragon
- Black pepper (ground), to taste

DIRECTIONS:

1) In a mixing bowl, whisk eggs and whites. Add cream cheese, milk, scallions, and tarragon. Combine to mix well with each other.

2) Take a medium saucepan or skillet, add butter. Heat over medium heat.

3) Add egg mixture and stir-cook for 4-5 minutes until eggs are scrambled evenly.
4) Season with black pepper and serve warm.

NUTRITION (Per Serving): Calories: 238; Fat: 17g; Phosphorus: 117mg; Potassium: 152mg; Sodium: 211mg; Carbohydrates: 3g; Protein: 8g.

Juice and Smoothies

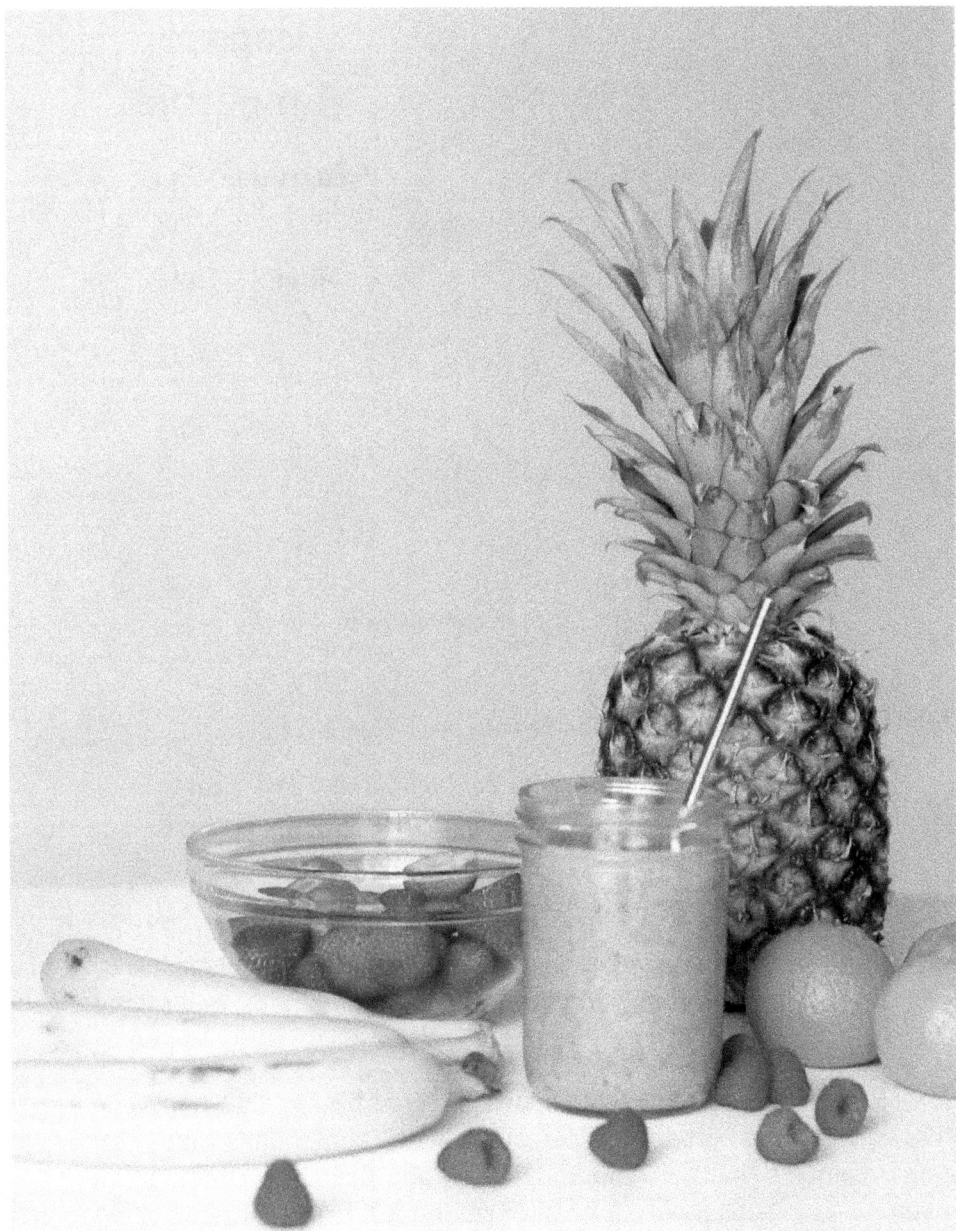

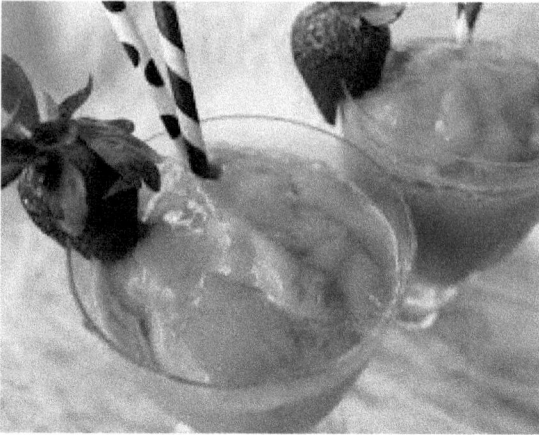

Strawberry Papaya Smoothie

Preparation Time: 10 minutes

Cooking Time: 0 minutes

Serving: 1

INGREDIENTS:

- ½ cup of strawberries
- 2 cups of sliced papaya
- 2 cup of coconut kefir
- 2 scoop of vanilla bone broth protein powder
- ½ cup of ice water

DIRECTIONS:

1) Add all of the ingredients to the blender and mix until the Strawberry Papaya Smoothie is pleasantly joined. I love including a crisp sprig of mint to supplement this new and fruity smoothie.

NUTRITION (Per Serving): Calories: 105; Fat: 19g; Phosphorus: 23mg; Potassium: 92mg; Sodium: 24mg; Carbohydrates: g; Protein: 2.8g.

EXTRA: Did you realize that papaya is incredible for digestion? The tropical organic product is stacked with compounds and cell reinforcements that help the body detox and decrease irritation. It's likewise a too delectable element for smoothies. In case you're hoping to switch your typical formula, it's a great opportunity to attempt this Strawberry Papaya Smoothie.

This beverage is without dairy and utilizes coconut kefir, a probiotic. When blended in with vanilla protein powder and crisp strawberries, you have a simple, hurried breakfast or post-exercise supper to fuel your body.

Cinnamon Egg Smoothie

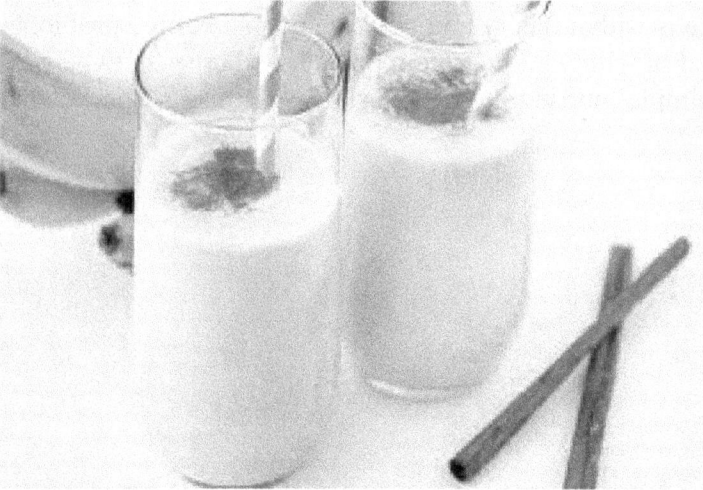

Preparation Time: 10 minutes

Cooking Time: 0 minutes

Serving: 1

INGREDIENTS:

- o   1/2 teaspoon ground cinnamon
- o   1 teaspoon stevia
- o   1/8 teaspoon vanilla extract
- o   8 oz. egg white, pasteurized
- o   3 tablespoons whipped topping

DIRECTIONS:

1) Mix the stevia, egg whites, cinnamon, and vanilla in a mixer.
2) Serve with whipped topping.
3) Enjoy.

NUTRITION (Per Serving): Calories 95; Total Fat 1.2g; Saturated Fat 0.6g; Cholesterol 3mg; Sodium 120mg; Carbohydrate 3.1g; Dietary Fiber 0.3g; Sugars 0.8g; Protein 12.5g; Calcium 18mg; Phosphorous 185mg; Potassium 194mg.

Pineapple Sorbet Smoothie

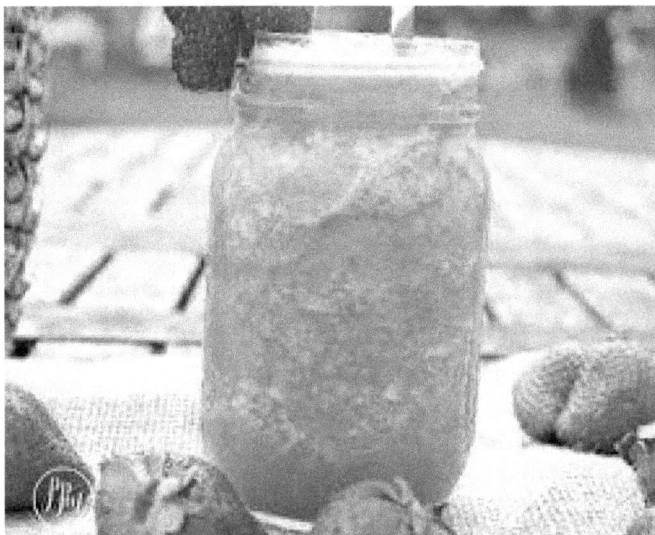

Preparation Time: 10 minutes

Cooking Time: 0 minutes

Serving: 1

INGREDIENTS:

- o   3/4 cup pineapple sorbet
- o   1 scoop protein powder
- o   1/2 cup water
- o   2 ice cubes, optional

DIRECTIONS:

1) First, begin by putting everything into a blender jug.
2) Pulse it for 30 seconds until well blended.
3) Serve chilled.

NUTRITION (Per Serving): Calories 180; Total Fat 1g; Saturated Fat 0.5g; Cholesterol 40mg; Sodium 86mg; Carbohydrate 30.5g; Dietary Fiber 0g; Sugars 28g; Protein 13g; Calcium 9mg; Phosphorous 164mg; Potassium 111mg.

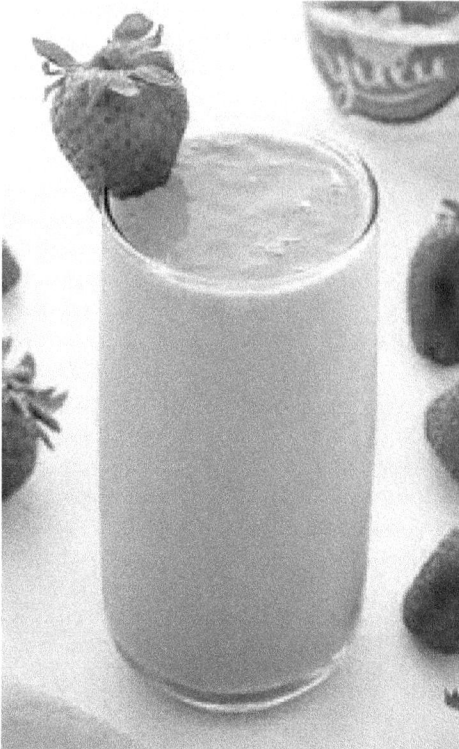

Vanilla Fruit Smoothie

Preparation Time: 10 minutes

Cooking Time: 0 minutes

Serving: 2

INGREDIENTS:

o   2 oz. mango, peeled and cubed
o   2 oz. strawberries
o   2 oz. avocado flesh, cubed
o   2 oz. banana, peeled
o   2 scoops of protein powder
o   1 cup cold water
o   1 cup crushed ice

DIRECTIONS:

1) First, begin by putting everything into a blender jug.
2) Pulse it for 30 seconds until well blended.
3) Serve chilled.

NUTRITION (Per Serving): Calories 228; Total Fat 7.6g; Saturated Fat 2.1g; Cholesterol 65mg; Sodium 58mg; Total Carbohydrate 19g; Dietary Fiber 3.6g; Sugars 9.8g; Protein 23.4g; Calcium 112mg; Phosphorous 216 mg; Potassium 504mg.

Cabbage and Chia Glass

Preparation Time: 10 minutes

Cooking Time: 30 minutes

Serving: 1

INGREDIENTS:

- 1/3 cup cabbage
- 1 cup cold unsweetened almond milk
- 1 tablespoon chia seeds
- ½ cup cherries
- ½ cup lettuce

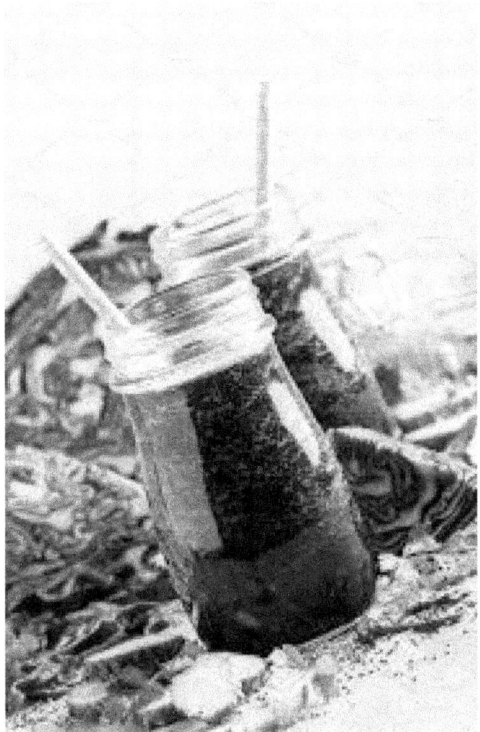

DIRECTIONS:

1) Add coconut milk to your blender.
2) Cut cabbage and add to your blender.
3) Place chia seeds in a coffee grinder and chop to powder, brush the powder into a blender.
4) Pit the cherries and add them to the blender.
5) Wash and dry the lettuce and chop.
6) Add to the mix.
7) Cover and blend on low followed by medium.
8) Taste the texture and serve chilled!

NUTRITION (Per Serving): Calories: 409; Phosphorus: 30mg; Potassium: 24mg; Sodium: 15mg; Fat: 33g; Carbohydrates: 8g; Protein: 12g.

Salads

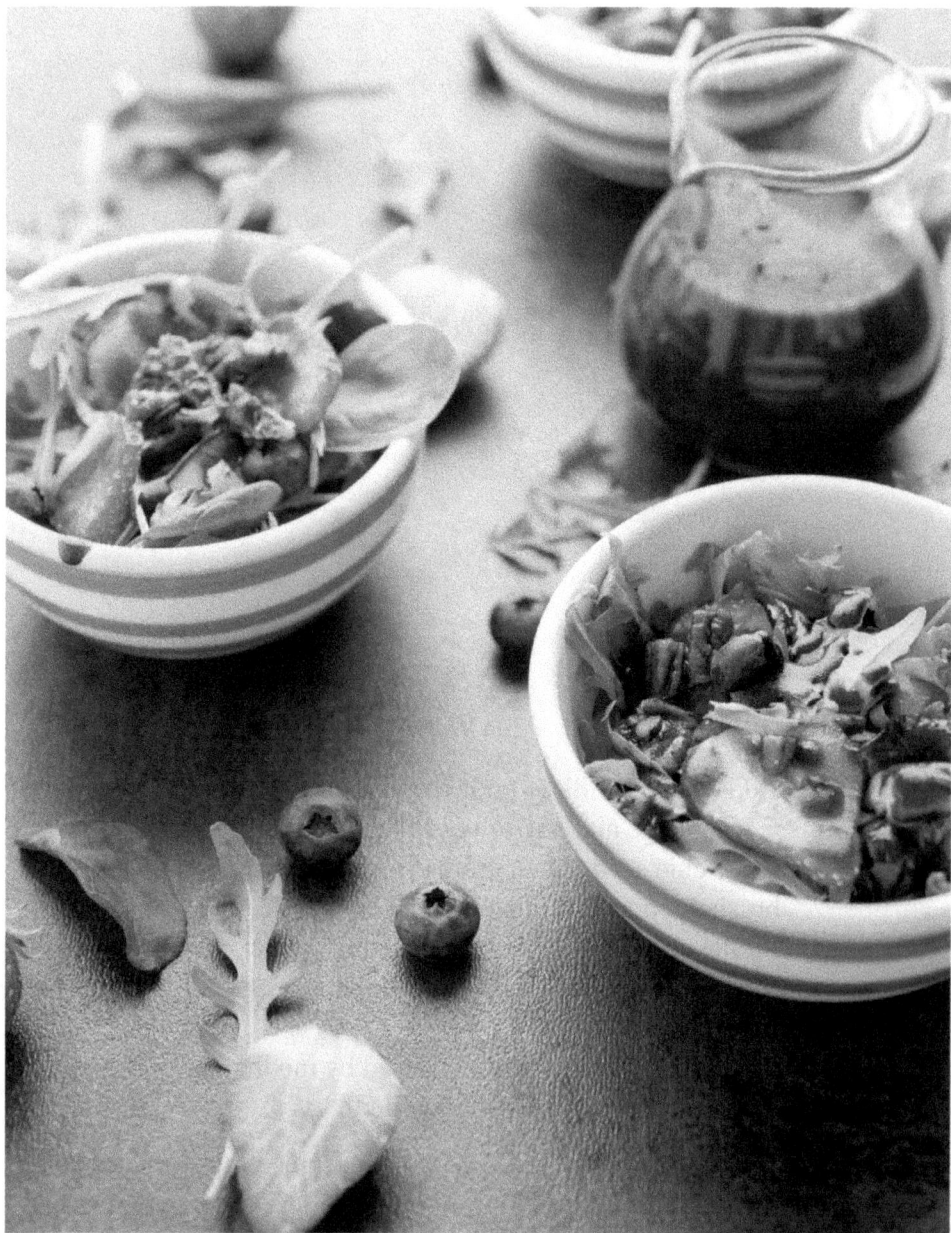

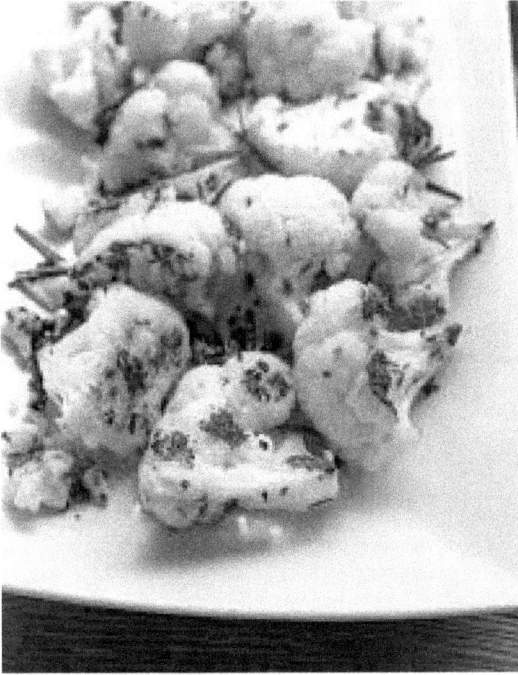

Rosemary and Roasted Cauliflower

Preparation Time: 10 minutes

Cooking Time: 30 minutes

Serving: 1

INGREDIENTS:

- o   1½ tablespoons olive oil
- o   1 medium head cauliflower
- o   ¼ teaspoon salt
- o   1 tablespoon fresh rosemary, finely chopped
- o   Fresh ground black pepper

DIRECTIONS:

1) Preheat oven to 450°F.
2) Cut florets from cauliflower head. Cut into bite-size pieces.
3) Toss the cauliflower with the rest of the ingredients in a large bowl.
4) Spread the seasoned cauliflower on an ungreased baking sheet.
5) Roast for 15 minutes. Remove from oven and stir.
6) Cook for 10 minutes until the cauliflower is tender.

NUTRITION (Per Serving): Protein - 1g; Phosphorus: 23mg; Potassium: 124mg; Sodium: 27mg; Carbohydrates - 2g; Fat - 2g; Calories – 32.

Roasted Wedges of Cabbage

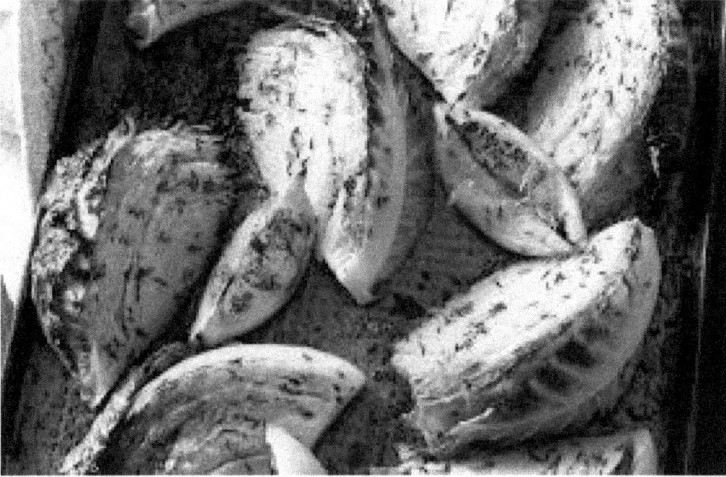

Preparation Time: 12 minutes

Cooking Time: 35 minutes

Serving: 2

INGREDIENTS:

- 2 teaspoon sugar
- 1 green cabbage, cut into 1-inch wedges
- 1 tablespoon balsamic vinegar
- ¼ teaspoon freshly ground pepper
- 2 tablespoon olive oil

DIRECTIONS:

1) Preheat oven to 450°F, with baking pan heating inside.
2) Combine sugar and pepper in a small bowl.
3) Brush cabbage wedges with oil. Sprinkle with pepper and sugar.
4) Put the seasoned wedges on the hot baking sheet. Roast until cabbage is browned and tender for 25 minutes.
5) Drizzle with balsamic vinegar.

NUTRITION (Per Serving): Protein - 0.74g; Phosphorus: 36mg; Potassium: 194mg; Sodium: 31mg; Carbohydrates - 4.0g; Fat - 1.8g; Calories - 32.3.

Green Bean Garlic Salad

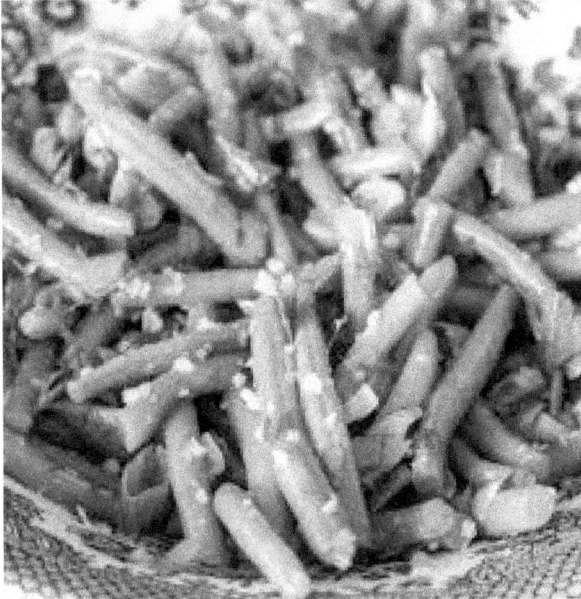

Preparation Time: 5 minutes

Cooking Time: 20 minutes

Serving: 2

INGREDIENTS:

- 2 cloves garlic, chopped
- 2 cups green beans
- 1 tablespoon sesame oil
- 1 tablespoon balsamic or red wine vinegar

DIRECTIONS:

1) Clean the beans. Cook them in boiling water until tender.
2) Drain and cool them under cold water.
3) Toss the beans with the oil, vinegar, and garlic.

NUTRITION (Per Serving): Protein - 1g; Phosphorus: 19mg; Potassium: 34mg; Sodium: 37mg; Carbohydrates - 6g; Fat - 4g; Calories – 59.

Beet Feta Salad

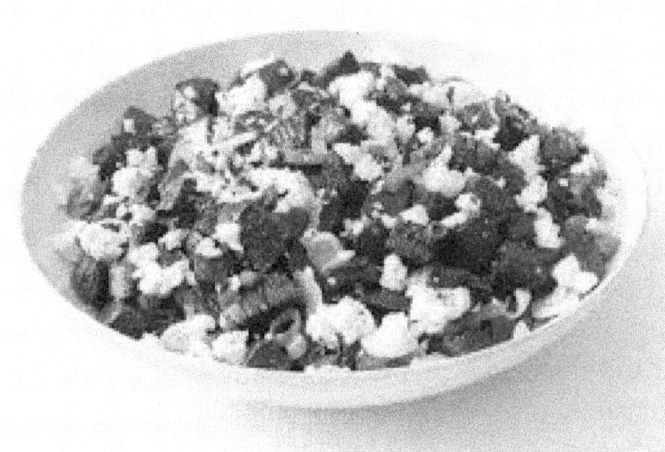

Preparation Time: 10 minutes

Cooking Time: 30 minutes

Serving: 2

INGREDIENTS:

- o 4 cups baby salad greens
- o ½ sweet onion, sliced
- o 8 small beets, trimmed
- o 2 tablespoons + 1 teaspoon extra-virgin olive oil
- o 1 tablespoon white wine vinegar
- o 1 teaspoon Dijon mustard
- o Black pepper (ground), to taste
- o 2 tablespoons crumbled feta cheese
- o 2 tablespoons walnut pieces

DIRECTIONS:

1) Preheat an oven to 400ºF. Grease an aluminum foil with some cooking spray.
2) Add beets with 1 teaspoon of olive oil; combine and wrap foil.
3) Bake for 30 minutes until it becomes tender. Cut beets into wedges.
4) In a mixing bowl, add remaining olive oil, vinegar, black pepper, and mustard. Combine to mix well with each other.
5) In a mixing bowl, add salad greens, onion, feta cheese, and walnuts. Combine to mix well with each other.
6) Add half of the prepared vinaigrette and toss well.
7) Add beet and combine well.
8) Drizzle remaining vinaigrette and serve fresh.

NUTRITION (Per Serving): Calories: 184; Fat: 9g; Phosphorus: 98mg; Potassium: 601mg; Sodium: 235mg; Carbohydrates: 19g; Protein: 4g.

Cucumber Salad

Preparation Time: 5 minutes

Cooking Time: 5 minutes

Serving: 2

INGREDIENTS:

- o   1 tablespoon dried dill
- o   1 onion
- o   ¼ cup water
- o   1 cup vinegar
- o   3 cucumbers
- o   ¾ cup white sugar

DIRECTIONS:

1) In a bowl add all ingredients and mix well.
2) Serve with dressing.

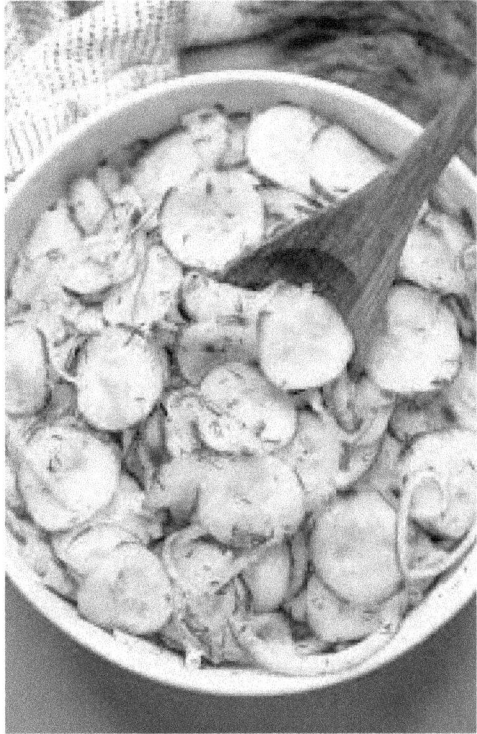

NUTRITION (Per Serving): Calories 49; Fat 0.1g; Sodium (Na) 341mg; Potassium (K) 171mg; Protein 0.8g; Carbs 11g; Phosphorus 24 mg.

Thai Cucumber Salad

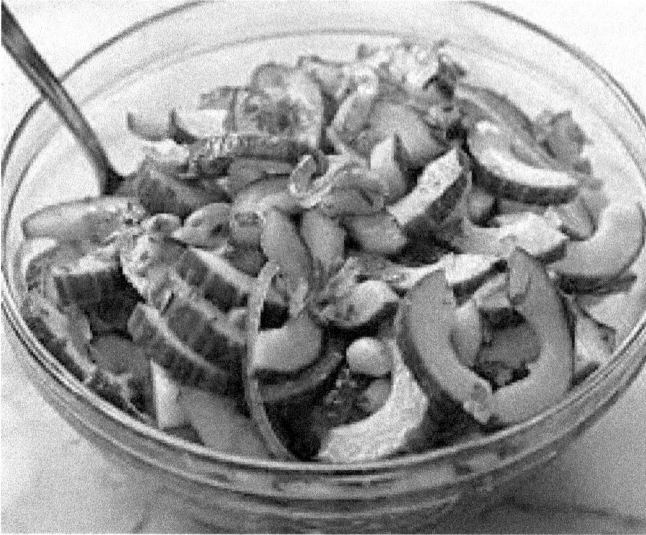

Preparation Time: 5 minutes

Cooking Time: 5 minutes

Serving: 2

INGREDIENTS:

- ¼ cup chopped peanuts
- ¼ cup white sugar
- ½ cup cilantro
- ¼ cup rice wine vinegar
- 3 cucumbers
- 2 jalapeno peppers

DIRECTIONS:

1) In a bowl add all ingredients and mix well.
2) Serve with dressing.

NUTRITION (Per Serving): Calories 20; Fat 0g; Sodium (Na) 85mg; Carbs 5g; Protein 1g; Potassium (K) 190.4 mg; Phosphorus 46.8mg.

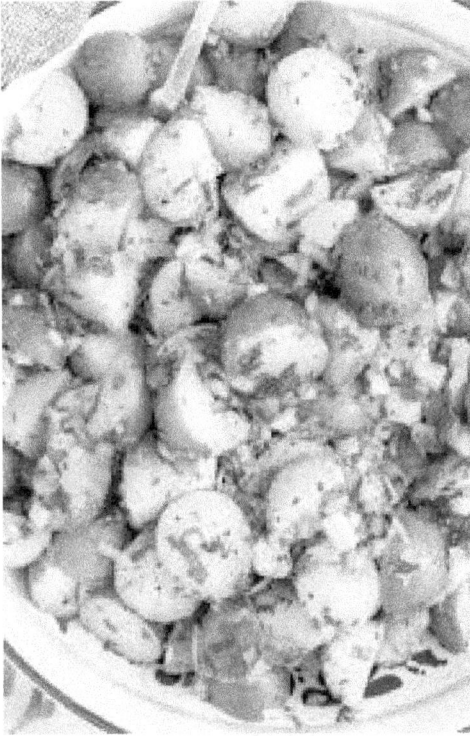

Red Potato Salad

Preparation Time: 5 minutes

Cooking Time: 5 minutes

Serving: 2

INGREDIENTS:

- 2 cups mayonnaise
- 1 lb. bacon
- 1 stalk celery
- 4 eggs
- Pepper
- 2 lbs. red potatoes
- 1 onion

DIRECTIONS:

1) In a pot add water, potatoes and cook until tender.
2) Remove, drain and set aside.
3) Place eggs in a saucepan, add water, and bring to a boil.
4) Cover and let eggs stand for 10-15 minutes.
5) When ready remove, meanwhile in a deep skillet cook bacon on low heat.
6) In a bowl add all ingredients and mix well.
7) Serve with dressing.

NUTRITION (Per Serving): Calories 280; Fat 20.0 g; Sodium (Na) 180.0 mg; Potassium (K) 0.0 mg; Carbs 26.0 g; Protein 2.0 g; Phosphorus 130mg

Soups and Stews

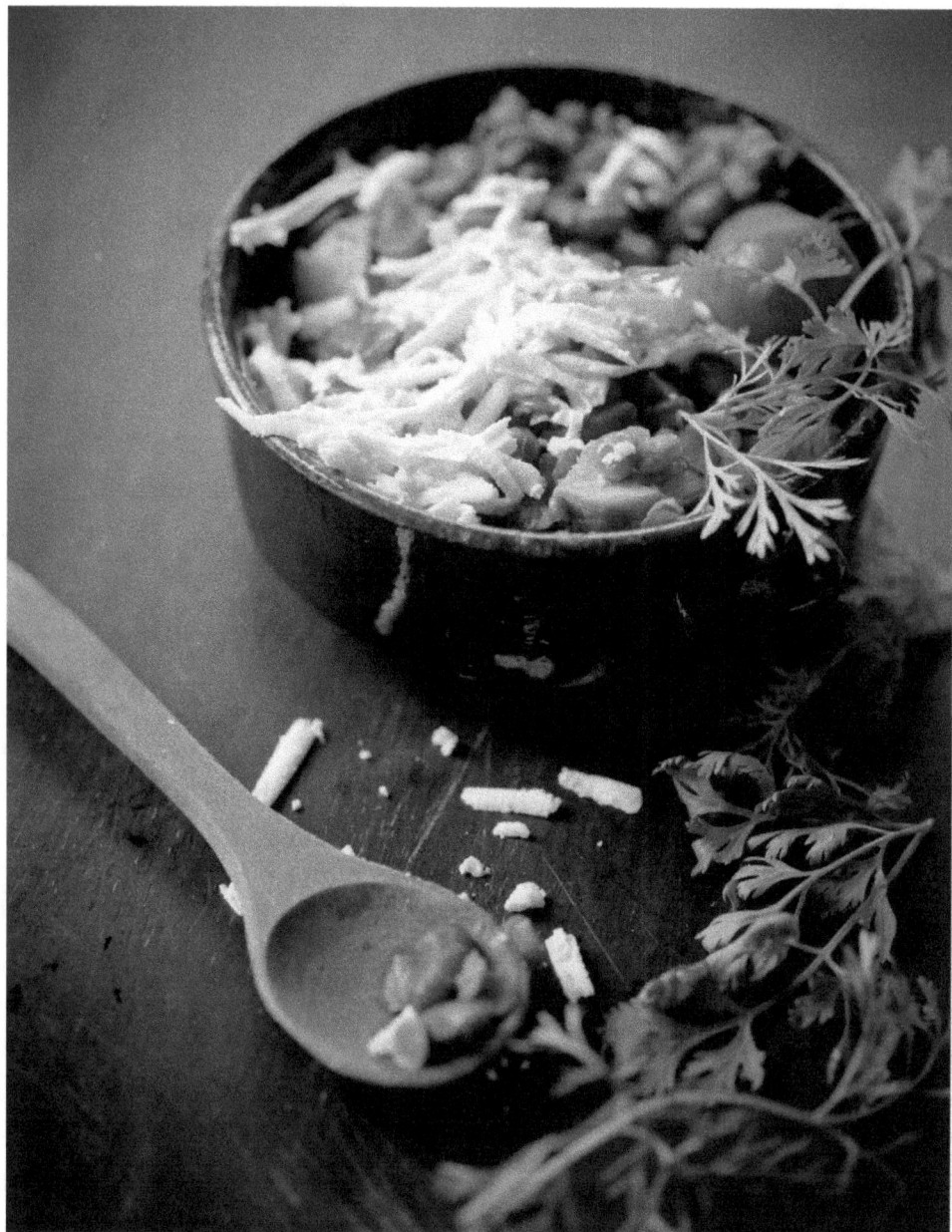

Classic Chicken Soup

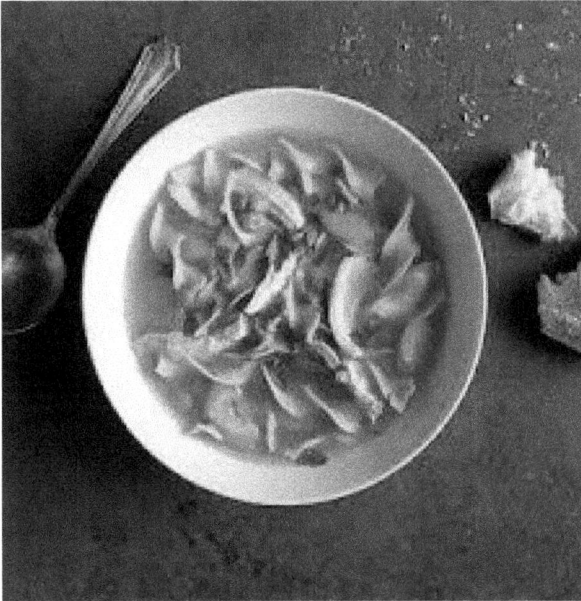

Preparation Time: 5-10 minutes

Cooking Time: 35 minutes

Serving: 1

INGREDIENTS:

- 2 teaspoons minced garlic
- 2 celery stalks, chopped
- 1 tablespoon unsalted butter
- ½ sweet onion, diced
- 1 carrot, diced
- 4 cups of water
- 1 teaspoon chopped fresh thyme
- 2 cups chopped cooked chicken breast
- 1 cup chicken stock
- Black pepper (ground), to taste
- 2 tablespoons chopped fresh parsley

DIRECTIONS:
1) Take a medium-large cooking pot, heat oil over medium heat.
2) Add onion and stir-cook until it becomes translucent and softened.
3) Add garlic and stir-cook until it becomes fragrant.
4) Add celery, carrot, chicken, chicken stock, and water.
5) Boil the mixture.
6) Over low heat, simmer the mixture for about 25-30 minutes until veggies are tender.
7) Mix in thyme and cook for 2 minutes. Season to taste with black pepper.
8) Serve warm with parsley on top.

NUTRITION (Per Serving): Calories: 135; Fat: 6g; Phosphorus: 122mg; Potassium: 208mg; Sodium: 74mg; Carbohydrates: 3g; Protein: 15g.

Beef Okra Soup

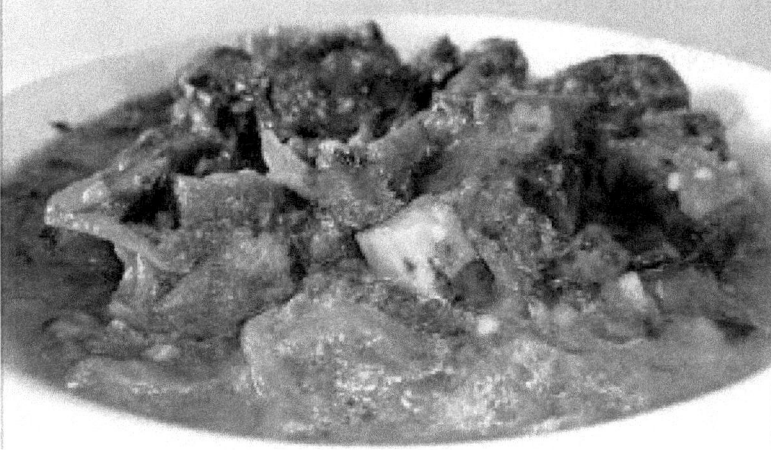

Preparation Time: 10 minutes

Cooking Time: 45-55 minutes

Serving: 1

INGREDIENTS:

- ½ cup okra
- ½ teaspoon basil
- ½ cup carrots, diced
- 3 ½ cups water
- 1-pound beef stew meat
- 1 cup raw sliced onions
- ½ cup green peas
- 1 teaspoon black pepper
- ½ teaspoon thyme
- ½ cup corn kernels

DIRECTIONS:

1) Take a medium-large cooking pot, heat oil over medium heat.
2) Add water, beef stew meat, black pepper, onions, basil, thyme, and stir-cook for 40-45 minutes until meat is tender.

3) Add all veggies. Over low heat, simmer the mixture for about 20-25 minutes. Add more water if needed.
4) Serve soup warm.

NUTRITION (Per Serving): Calories: 187; Fat: 12g; Phosphorus: 119mg; Potassium: 288mg; Sodium: 59mg; Carbohydrates: 7g; Protein: 11g.

Green Bean Veggie Stew

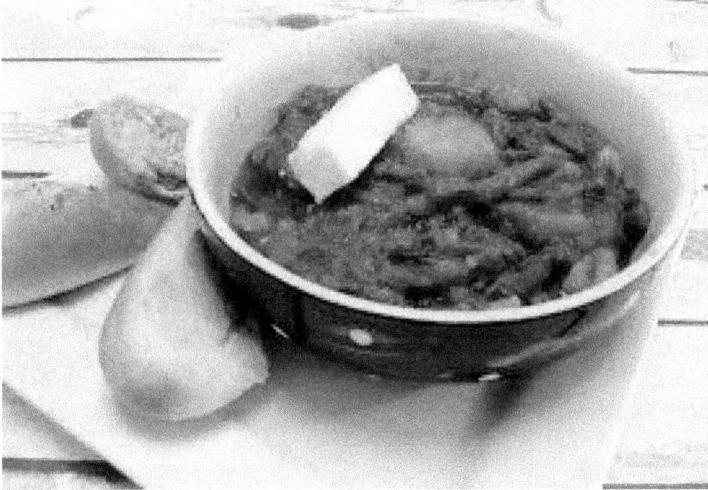

Preparation Time: 10 minutes

Cooking Time:30-35 minutes

Serving: 1

INGREDIENTS:

- o   6 cups shredded green cabbage
- o   3 celery stalks, chopped
- o   1 teaspoon unsalted butter
- o   ½ large sweet onion, chopped
- o   1 teaspoon minced garlic
- o   1 scallion, chopped
- o   2 tablespoons chopped fresh parsley
- o   2 tablespoons lemon juice
- o   1 teaspoon chopped fresh oregano
- o   1 tablespoon chopped fresh thyme
- o   1 teaspoon chopped savory
- o   Water
- o   1 cup fresh green beans, cut into 1-inch pieces
- o   Black pepper (ground), to taste

DIRECTIONS:

1) Take a medium-large cooking pot, heat butter over medium heat.
2) Add onion and stir-cook until it becomes translucent and soft.
3) Add garlic and stir-cook until it becomes fragrant.
4) Add cabbage, celery, scallion, parsley, lemon juice, thyme, savory, and oregano; add water to cover veggies by 3-4 inches.
5) Stir the mixture and boil it.
6) Over low heat, cover, and simmer the mixture for about 25 minutes until veggies are tender.
7) Add green beans and cook for 2-3 more minutes. Season with black pepper to taste.
8) Serve warm.

NUTRITION (Per Serving): Calories: 56; Fat: 1g; Phosphorus: 36mg; Potassium: 194mg; Sodium: 31mg; Carbohydrates: 7g; Protein: 1g.

Chicken Pasta Soup

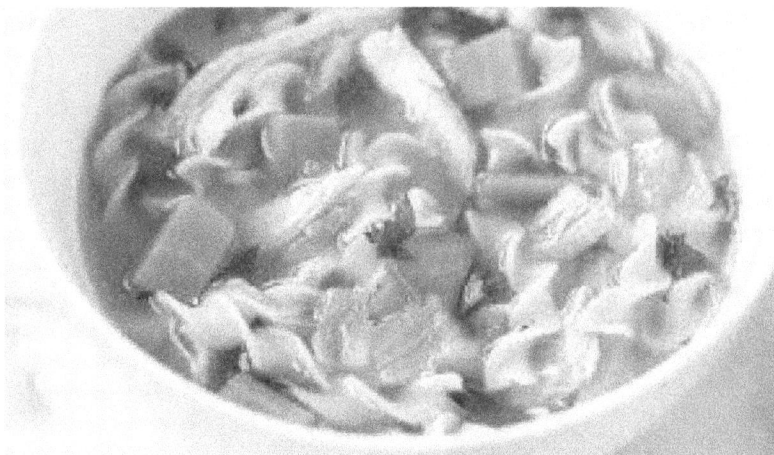

Preparation Time: 10 minutes

Cooking Time: 20 minutes

Serving: 1

INGREDIENTS:
- 1 ½ cups baby spinach
- 2 tablespoons orzo (tiny pasta)
- 1 tablespoon dry white wine
- 1 14-ounce low sodium chicken broth
- 2 plum tomatoes, chopped
- ½ teaspoon Italian seasoning
- 1 large shallot, chopped
- 1 small zucchini, diced
- 8-ounces chicken tenders
- 1 tablespoon extra-virgin olive oil

DIRECTIONS:
1) Take a medium saucepan or skillet, add oil. Heat over medium heat.
2) Add chicken and stir-cook for 3 minutes until evenly brown. Set aside.

3) In the pan, add zucchini, Italian seasoning, shallot; stir-cook until veggies are softened.
4) Add tomatoes, wine, broth, and orzo.
5) Boil the mixture.
6) Over low heat, cover, and simmer the mixture for about 3 minutes.
7) Mix in spinach and cooked chicken; stir and serve warm.

NUTRITION (Per Serving): Calories: 103; Fat: 3g; Phosphorus: 125mg; Potassium: 264mg; Sodium: 84mg; Carbohydrates: 6g; Protein: 12g.

Fish and Seafood

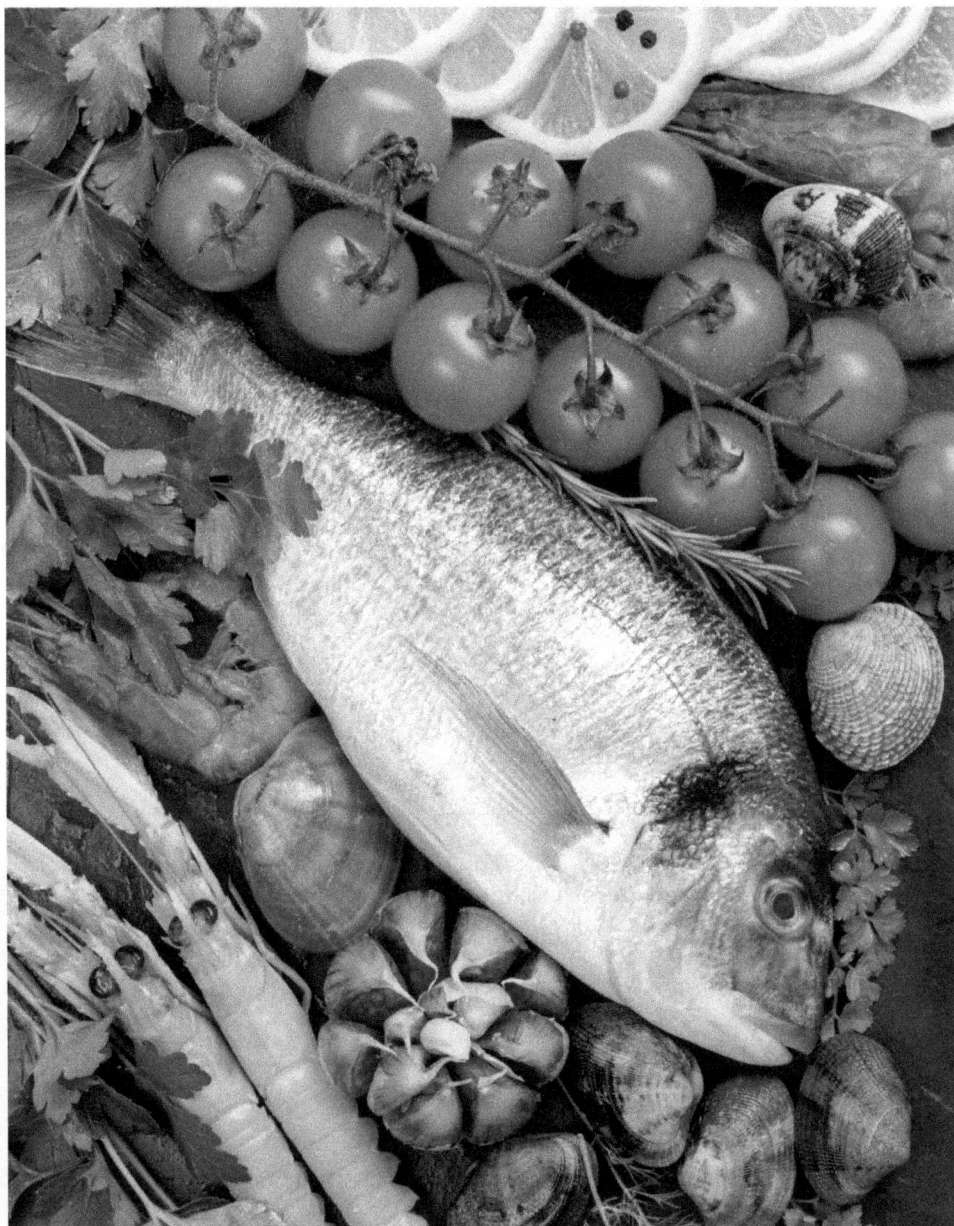

Lemony Haddock

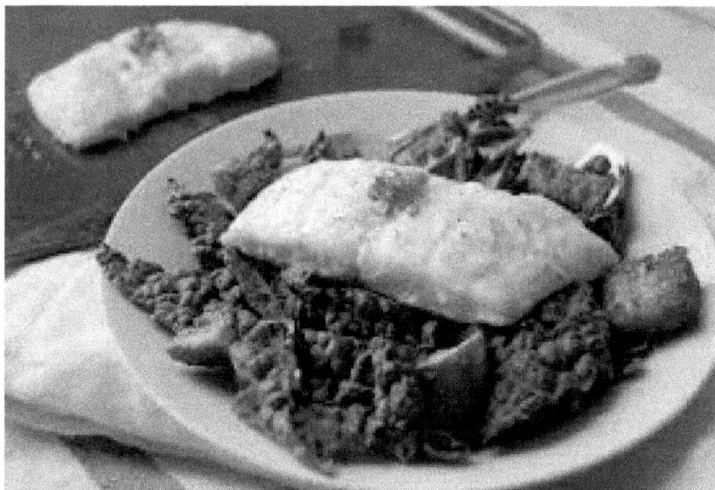

Preparation Time: 10 minutes

Cooking Time: 20 minutes

Serving: 1

INGREDIENTS:

- o 1 tablespoon melted unsalted butter
- o 12-ounces haddock fillets, deboned and skinned
- o ½ cup breadcrumbs
- o 3 tablespoons chopped fresh parsley
- o 1 tablespoon lemon zest
- o 1 teaspoon chopped fresh thyme
- o ¼ teaspoon black pepper (ground)

DIRECTIONS:

1) Preheat the oven to 350ºF.
2) In a mixing bowl, add breadcrumbs, parsley, lemon zest, thyme, and pepper. Combine to mix well.
3) Add butter and combine until you get crumbles.

4) Take a baking sheet and place haddock on it. Add crumb mixture on top.
5) Bake for 18-20 minutes until evenly brown from top.
6) Serve warm.

NUTRITION (Per Serving): Calories: 183; Fat: 4g; Phosphorus: 233mg; Potassium: 305mg; Sodium: 316mg; Carbohydrates: 9g; Protein: 16g.

Glazed Salmon

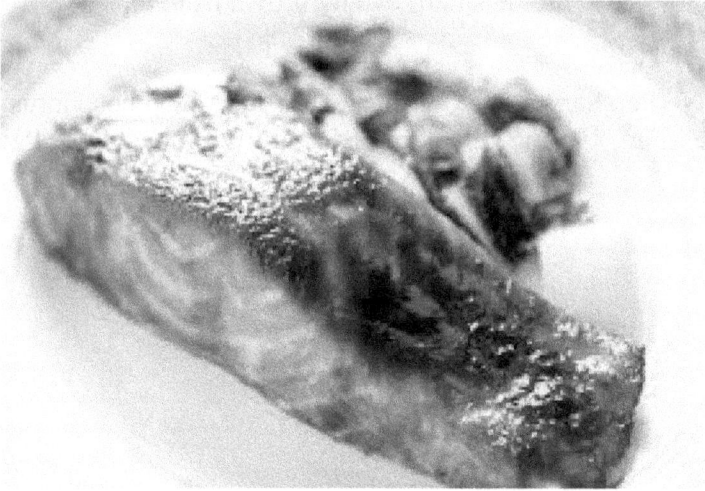

Preparation Time: 10 minutes

Cooking Time: 10 minutes

Serving: 1

INGREDIENTS:

- o   4 (3-ounce) salmon fillets
- o   1 tablespoon olive oil
- o   2 tablespoons honey
- o   1 teaspoon lemon zest
- o   ½ teaspoon Black pepper (ground), to taste
- o   ½ scallion, chopped

DIRECTIONS:

1) Pat dry salmon with paper towels.
2) In a mixing bowl, add honey, lemon zest, and pepper. Combine to mix well.
3) Add salmon and coat evenly.
4) Take a medium saucepan or skillet, add oil. Heat over medium heat.

5) Add salmon and stir-cook until light brown and cooked well, for about 8-10 minutes. Flip in between.
6) Serve warm with scallions on top.

NUTRITION (Per Serving): Calories: 238; Fat: 13g; Phosphorus: 220mg; Potassium: 348mg; Sodium: 74mg; Carbohydrates: 10g; Protein: 16g.

Tuna Casserole

Preparation Time: 15 minutes

Cooking Time: 35 minutes

Serving: 1

INGREDIENTS:

- ½ cup Cheddar cheese, shredded
- 2 tomatoes, chopped
- 7 oz tuna filet, chopped
- 1 teaspoon ground coriander
- ½ teaspoon salt
- 1 teaspoon olive oil
- ½ teaspoon dried oregano

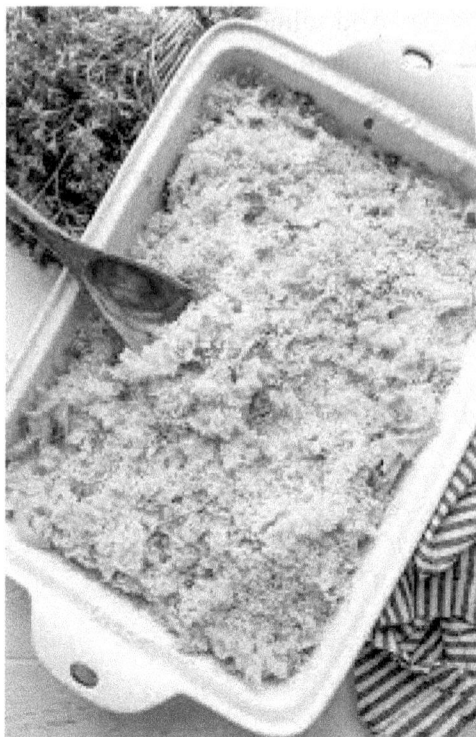

DIRECTIONS:

1) Brush the casserole mold with olive oil.
2) Mix together chopped tuna fillet with dried oregano and ground coriander.
3) Place the fish in the mold and flatten well to get the layer.
4) Then add chopped tomatoes and shredded cheese.
5) Cover the casserole with foil and secure the edges.
6) Bake the meal for 35 minutes at 355^0 F.

NUTRITION (Per Serving): Calories 260; Fat 21.5; Phosphorus: 56mg; Potassium: 64mg; Sodium: 29mg; Fiber 0.8; Carbs 2.7; Protein 14.6.

Oregano Salmon with Crunchy Crust

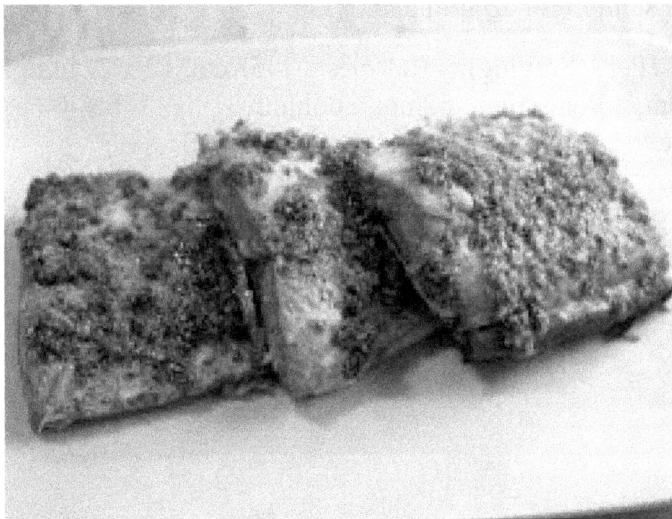

Preparation Time: 10 minutes

Cooking Time: 2 hours

Serving: 2

INGREDIENTS:

- o   8 oz salmon fillet
- o   2 tablespoons panko breadcrumbs
- o   1 oz Parmesan, grated
- o   1 teaspoon dried oregano
- o   1 teaspoon sunflower oil

DIRECTIONS:

1) In the mixing bowl combine panko breadcrumbs, Parmesan, and dried oregano.
2) Sprinkle the salmon with olive oil and coat in the breadcrumb's mixture.
3) After this, line the baking tray with baking paper.

4) Place the salmon in the tray and transfer to the oven preheated at 385^0 F.
5) Bake the salmon for 25 minutes.

NUTRITION (Per Serving): Calories 245Kcal; Fat 12.8g; Phosphorus: 30mg; Potassium: 67mg; Sodium: 31mg; Fiber 0.6g; Carbs 5.9g; Protein 27.5g.

Sardine Fish Cakes

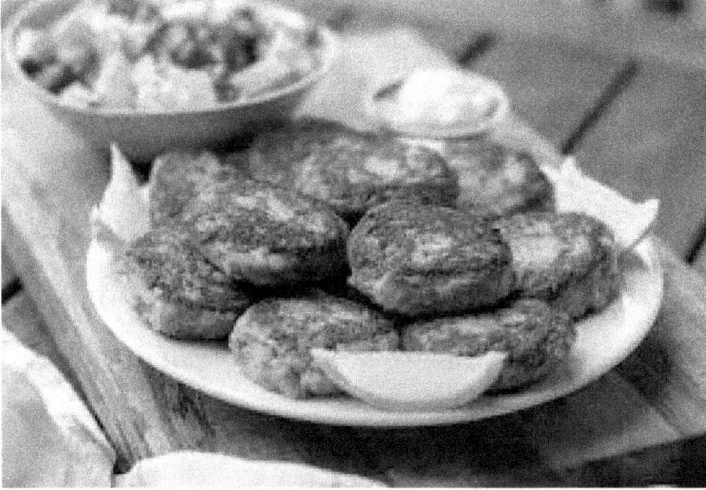

Preparation Time: 10 minutes

Cooking Time: 10 minutes

Serving: 1

INGREDIENTS:

- o   11 oz sardines, canned, drained
- o   1/3 cup shallot, chopped
- o   1 teaspoon chili flakes
- o   ½ teaspoon salt
- o   2 tablespoon wheat flour, whole grain
- o   1 egg, beaten
- o   1 tablespoon chives, chopped
- o   1 teaspoon olive oil
- o   1 teaspoon butter

DIRECTIONS:

1) Put the butter in the skillet and melt it.
2) Add shallot and cook it until translucent.
3) After this, transfer the shallot in the mixing bowl.
4) Add sardines, chili flakes, salt, flour, egg, chives, and mix up until smooth with the help of the fork.
5) Make the medium size cakes and place them in the skillet.
6) Add olive oil.
7) Roast the fish cakes for 3 minutes from each side over the medium heat.
8) Dry the cooked fish cakes with the paper towel if needed and transfer in the serving plates.

NUTRITION (Per Serving): Calories 221; Fat 12.2; Phosphorus: 36mg; Potassium: 194mg; Sodium: 31mg; Fiber 0.1; Carbs 5.4; Protein 21.3

Cajun Catfish

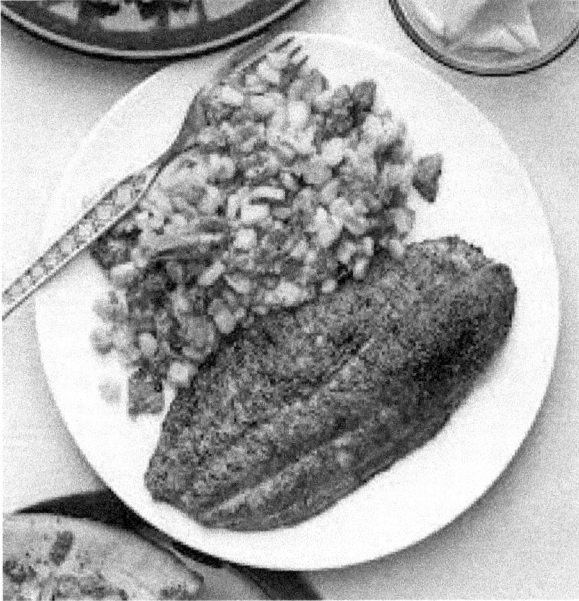

Preparation Time: 10 minutes

Cooking Time: 10 minutes

Serving: 1

INGREDIENTS:

- 16 oz catfish steaks (4 oz each fish steak)
- 1 tablespoon Cajun spices
- 1 egg, beaten
- 1 tablespoon sunflower oil

DIRECTIONS:

1) Heat oil in a pan.
2) Meanwhile, dip every catfish steak in the beaten egg and coat in Cajun spices.
3) Place the fish steaks in the hot oil and roast them for 4 minutes from each side.

4) The cooked catfish steaks should have a light brown crust.

NUTRITION (Per Serving): Calories 263; Fat 16.7; Phosphorus: 39mg; Potassium: 74mg; Sodium: 20mg; Fiber 0; Carbs 0.1; Protein 26.3.

Meat

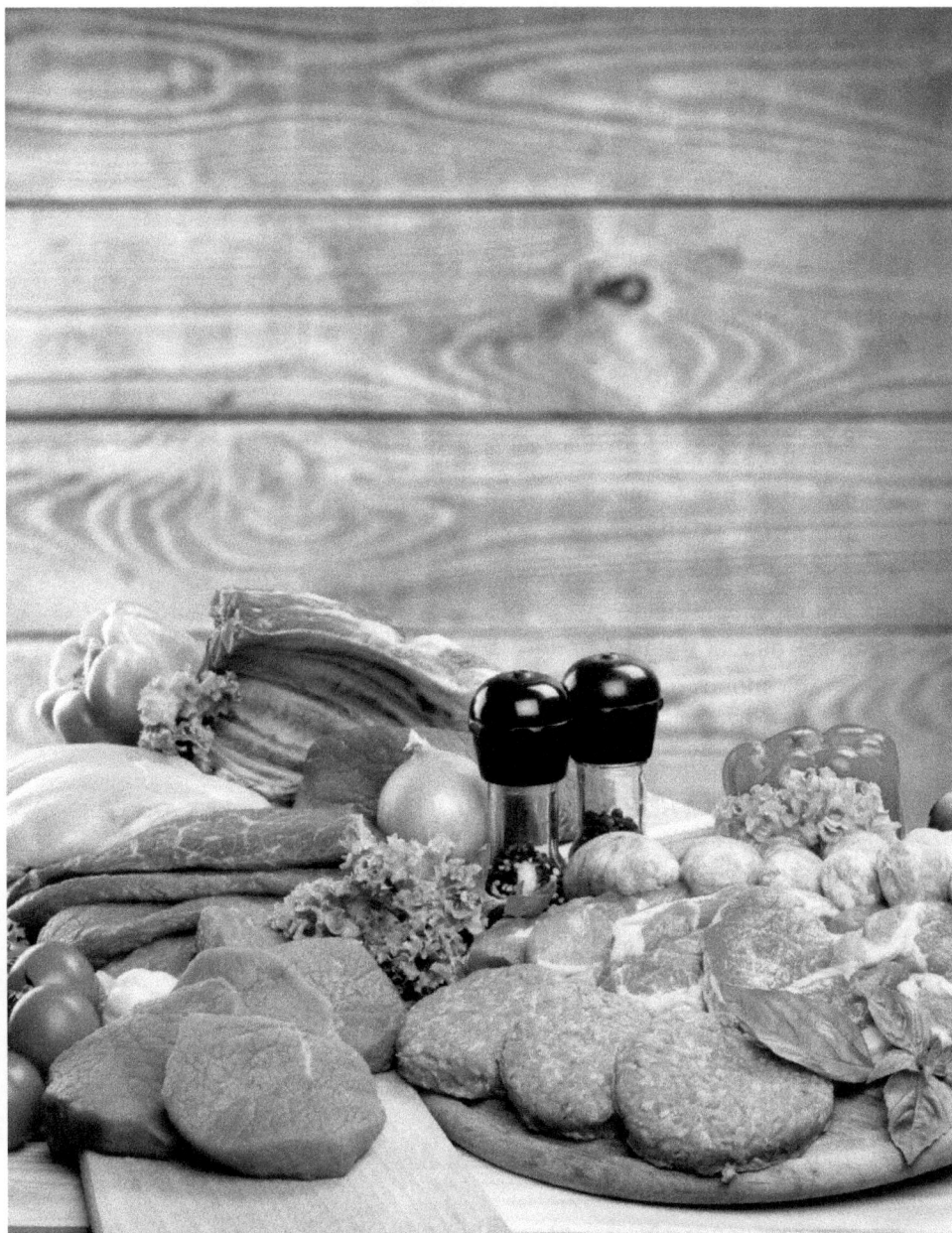

Beef Stew with Apple Cider

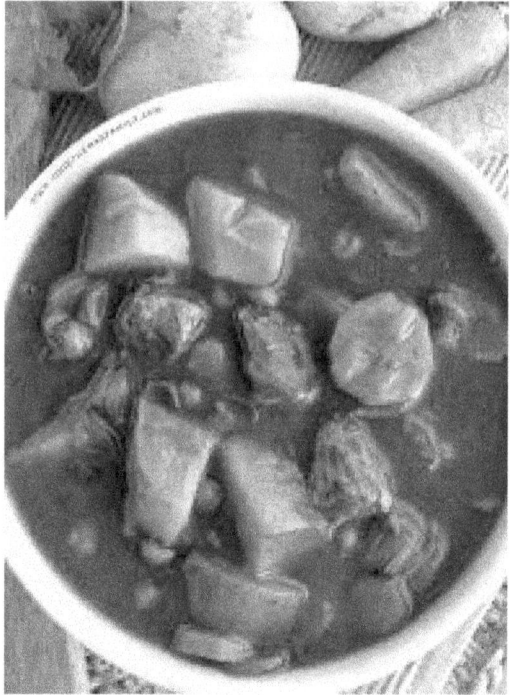

Preparation Time: 15 minutes

Cooking Time: 10 hours

Serving: 2

INGREDIENTS:

- o 1/2 cup potatoes, cubed
- o 2 lb. beef cubes
- o 7 tablespoons all-purpose flour, divided
- o 1/4 teaspoon thyme
- o Black pepper to taste
- o 3 tablespoons oil
- o ¼ cup carrot, sliced
- o 1 cup onion, diced
- o 1/2 cup celery, diced
- o 1 cup apples, diced
- o 2 cups apple cider
- o 1/2 cups water
- o 2 tablespoons apple cider vinegar

DIRECTIONS:

1) Double boil the potatoes (to reduce the amount of potassium) in a pot of water.
2) In a shallow dish, mix the half of the flour, thyme, and pepper.
3) Coat all sides of beef cubes with the mixture.

4) In a pan, add the oil over medium heat, and cook the beef cubes until brown. Set aside.
5) Layer the ingredients in your slow cooker.
6) Put the carrots, potatoes, onions, celery, beef, and apple.
7) In a bowl, mix the cider, vinegar, and 1cup of water.
8) Add this to the slow cooker.
9) Cook on low setting for 10 hours.
10) Stir in the remaining flour to thicken the soup.

NUTRITION (Per Serving): Calories 365; Protein 33 g; Carbohydrates 20 g; Fat 17 g; Cholesterol 73 mg; Sodium 80 mg; Potassium 540 mg; Phosphorus 234 mg; Calcium 36 mg; Fiber 2.2 g.

Steak Burgers/Sandwich

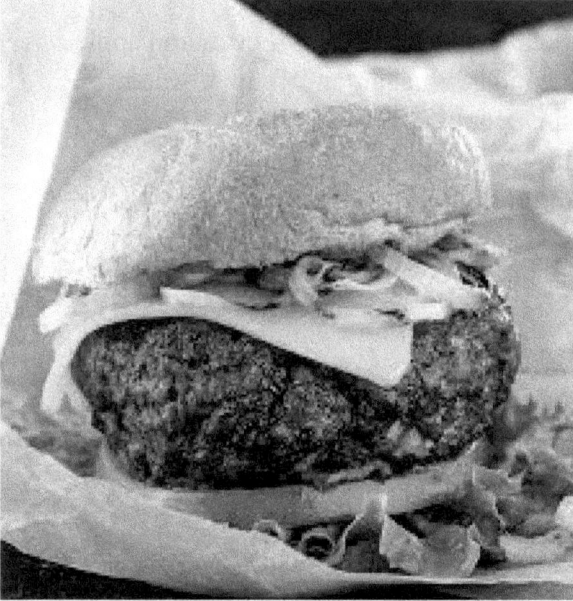

Preparation Time: 10 minutes

Cooking Time: 8-10 minutes

Serving: 1

INGREDIENTS:

- o 1 tablespoon lemon juice
- o 1 tablespoon Italian seasoning
- o 1 teaspoon black pepper
- o 4 flank steaks (around 4 oz. each)
- o 1 medium red onion, sliced
- o 1 tablespoon vegetable oil
- o 4 sandwich/burger buns

DIRECTIONS:

1) Season steaks with lemon juice, Italian seasoning, and black pepper.
2) Take a medium saucepan or skillet, add oil. Heat over medium heat.
3) Add steaks and stir-cook for 5-6 minutes until evenly brown. Set aside.
4) Add onion and stir-cook for 2-3 minutes until it becomes translucent and softened.
5) Slice burger buns into half and place 1 steak piece over.
6) Add onion mixture on top. Add another bun piece on top and serve fresh.

NUTRITION (Per Serving): Calories: 349; Fat: 12g; Phosphorus: 312mg; Potassium: 241mg; Sodium: 287mg; Carbohydrates: 9g; Protein: 36g.

Broiled Lamb Shoulder

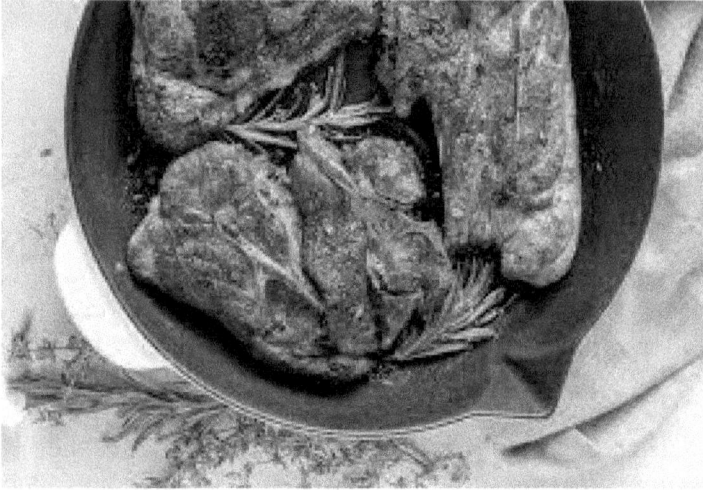

Preparation Time: 10 minutes

Cooking Time: 8-10 minutes

Serving: 1

INGREDIENTS:

- o 2 tablespoons fresh ginger, minced
- o 2 tablespoons garlic, minced
- o ¼ cup fresh lemongrass stalk, minced
- o ¼ cup fresh orange juice
- o ¼ cup coconut aminos
- o Freshly ground black pepper, to taste
- o 2-pound lamb shoulder, trimmed

DIRECTIONS:

1) In a bowl, mix all ingredients except lamb shoulder.
2) In a baking dish, squeeze lamb shoulder and coat the lamb with half of the marinade mixture generously.
3) Reserve remaining mixture.
4) Refrigerate to marinate overnight.

5) Preheat the broiler of the oven. Place a rack inside a broiler pan and arrange about 4-5-inches from the heating unit.
6) Remove the lamb shoulder from the refrigerator and remove excess marinade.
7) Broil approximately 4-5 minutes from both sides.
8) Serve with all the reserved marinade like a sauce.

NUTRITION (Per Serving): Calories: 250; Fat: 19g; Phosphorus: 46mg; Potassium: 84mg; Sodium: 29mg; Carbohydrates: 2g; Fiber: 0g; Protein: 15g.

Pan-Seared Lamb Chops

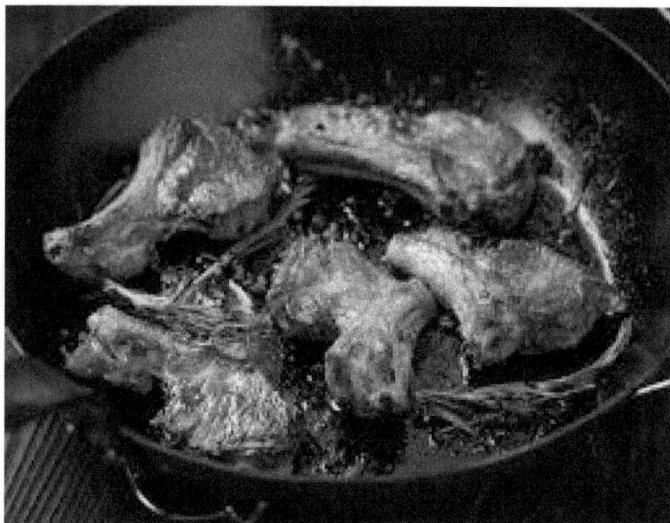

Preparation Time: 10 minutes

Cooking Time: 4-6 minutes

Serving: 1

INGREDIENTS:

- 4 garlic cloves, peeled
- Salt, to taste
- 1 teaspoon black mustard seeds, crushed finely
- 2 teaspoons ground cumin
- 1 teaspoon ground ginger
- 1 teaspoon ground coriander
- ½ teaspoon ground cinnamon
- Freshly ground black pepper, to taste
- 1 tablespoon coconut oil
- 8 medium lamb chops, trimmed

DIRECTIONS:

1) Place garlic cloves onto a cutting board and sprinkle with salt.
2) With a knife, crush the garlic till a paste form.
3) In a bowl, mix garlic paste and spices.
4) With a clear, crisp knife, make 3-4 cuts on both sides in the chops.
5) Rub the chops with garlic mixture generously.
6) In a large skillet, melt butter on medium heat.
7) Add chops and cook for approximately 2-3 minutes per side or till the desired doneness.

NUTRITION (Per Serving): Calories: 443; Fat: 11g; Phosphorus: 36mg; Potassium: 64mg; Sodium: 24mg; Carbohydrates: 27g; Fiber: 4g; Protein: 40g.

Roasted Lamb Chops with Relish

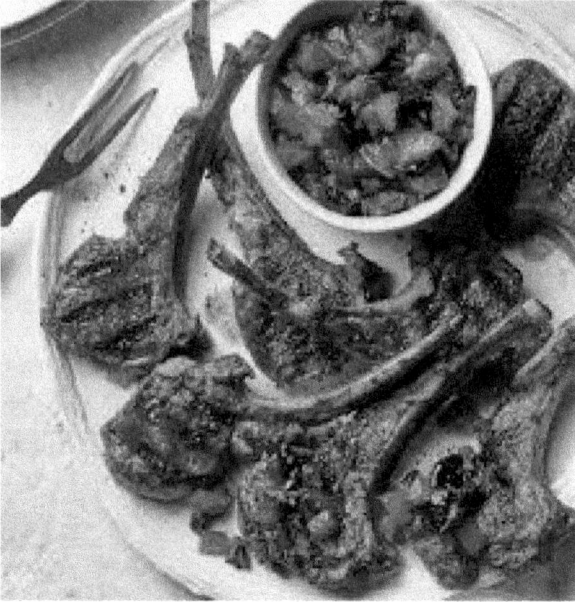

Preparation Time: 15 minutes

Cooking Time: 30 minutes

Serving: 1

INGREDIENTS:

For Lamb Marinade:

- o 4 garlic cloves, chopped
- o 1 (2-inch) piece fresh ginger, chopped
- o 2 green chilies, seeded and chopped
- o 1 teaspoon fresh lime zest
- o 2 teaspoons garam masala
- o 1 teaspoon ground coriander
- o 1 teaspoon ground cumin
- o ½ teaspoon ground cinnamon
- o 1 teaspoon coconut oil, melted
- o 2 tablespoons fresh lime juice

- o 6-7 tablespoons plain Greek yogurt
- o 1 (8-bone) rack of lamb, trimmed
- o 2 onions, sliced

For Relish:

- o ½ of garlic herb, chopped
- o 1 (1-inch) piece fresh ginger, chopped
- o ¼ cup fresh cilantro, chopped
- o ¼ cup fresh mint, chopped
- o 1 green chili, seeded and chopped
- o 1 teaspoon fresh lime zest
- o 1 teaspoon organic honey
- o 2 tablespoons fresh apple juice
- o 2 tablespoons fresh lime juice

DIRECTIONS:

1) For chops marinade, in a mixer, add all ingredients except yogurt, chops, and onions and pulse till smooth.
2) Transfer the mixture in a large bowl with yogurt and stir to combine well.
3) Add chops and coat them generously with the mixture.
4) Refrigerate to marinate for approximately 24 hours.
5) Preheat the oven to 375^0 F. Line a roasting pan with a foil paper.
6) Place the onion wedges in the bottom of the prepared roasting pan.
7) Arrange rack of lamb over onion wedges.
8) Roast approximately for 30 minutes.
9) Meanwhile, for relish, in the blender, add all ingredients and pulse till smooth.
10) Serve chops and onions alongside relish.

NUTRITION (Per Serving): Calories: 439; Fat: 17g; Phosphorus: 45mg; Potassium: 156mg; Sodium: 30mg; Carbohydrates: 26g; Fiber: 10g; Protein: 41g.

Grilled Lamb Chops

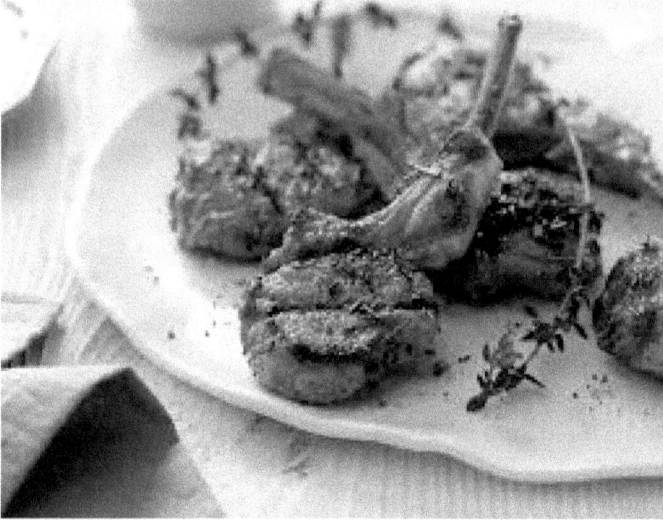

Preparation Time: 10 minutes

Cooking Time: 6 minutes

Serving: 1

INGREDIENTS:

- 1 tablespoon fresh ginger, grated
- 4 garlic cloves, chopped roughly
- 1 teaspoon ground cumin
- ½ teaspoon red chili powder
- Salt and freshly ground black pepper, to taste
- 1 tablespoon essential olive oil
- 1 tablespoon fresh lemon juice
- 8 lamb chops, trimmed

DIRECTIONS:

1) In a bowl, mix all ingredients except chops.
2) With a hand blender, blend till a smooth mixture is formed.
3) Add chops and coat generously with mixture.

4) Refrigerate to marinate overnight.
5) Preheat the barbecue grill till hot. Grease the grill grate.
6) Grill the chops for approximately 3 minutes per side.
7) Serve when done.

NUTRITION (Per Serving): Calories: 227; Fat: 12g; Phosphorus: 36mg; Potassium: 194mg; Sodium: 31mg; Carbohydrates: 1g; Fiber: 0g; Protein: 30g.

Lamb Burgers with Avocado Dip

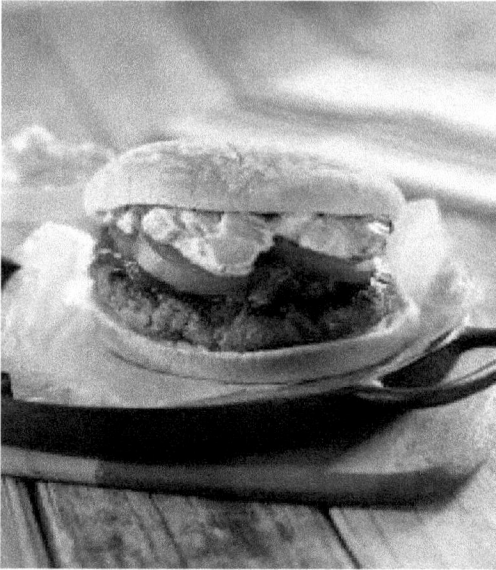

Preparation Time: 20 minutes

Cooking Time: 10 minutes

Serving: 1

INGREDIENTS:

For Burgers:

- o   1 (2-inch) piece fresh ginger, grated
- o   1-pound lean ground lamb
- o   1 medium onion, grated
- o   2 minced garlic cloves
- o   1 bunch fresh mint leaves, chopped finely
- o   2 teaspoons ground coriander
- o   2 teaspoons ground cumin
- o   ½ teaspoon ground allspice
- o   ½ teaspoon ground cinnamon
- o   Salt and freshly ground black pepper, to taste
- o   1 tablespoon essential olive oil

For Dip:

- o 3 small cucumbers, peeled and grated
- o 1 avocado, peeled, pitted, and chopped
- o ½ of garlic oil, crushed
- o 2 tablespoons fresh lemon juice
- o 2 tablespoons olive oil
- o 2 tablespoons fresh dill, chopped finely
- o 2 tablespoons chives, chopped finely
- o Salt and freshly ground black pepper, to taste

DIRECTIONS:

1) Preheat the broiler of the oven. Lightly, grease a broiler pan.
2) For burgers in a big bowl, squeeze the juice of ginger.
3) Add remaining ingredients and mix till well combined.
4) Make equal sized burgers patties from your mixture.
5) Arrange the burgers patties in the broiler pan and broil approximately 5 minutes per side.
6) Meanwhile, for dip squeeze the cucumbers juice in a bowl.
7) In a blender, add avocado, garlic, lemon juice, and oil and pulse till smooth.
8) Transfer the avocado mixture into a bowl.
9) Add remaining ingredients and stir to mix.
10) Assemble the burger and serve them with avocado dip.

NUTRITION (Per Serving): Calories: 462; Fat: 15g; Phosphorus: 32mg; Potassium: 178mg; Sodium 56mg; Carbohydrates: 23g; Fiber: 9g; Protein: 39g.

Lamb & Pineapple Kebabs

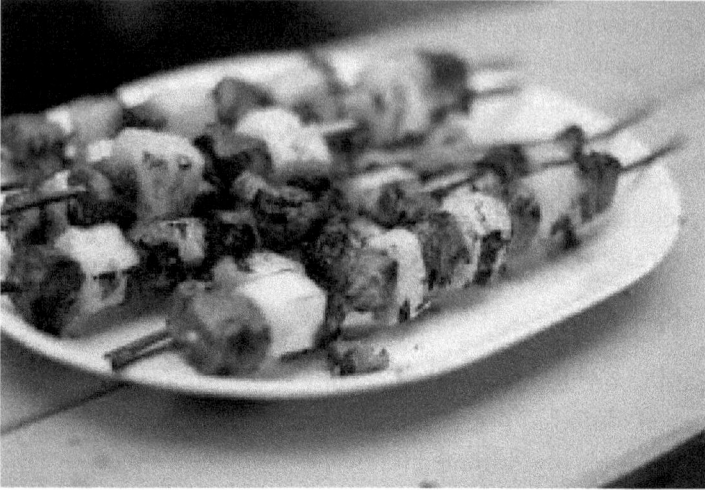

Preparation Time: 15 minutes

Cooking Time: 10 minutes

Serving: 1

INGREDIENTS:

- 1 large pineapple, cubed into 1½-inch size, divided
- 1 (½-inch) piece fresh ginger, chopped
- 2 garlic cloves, chopped
- Salt, to taste
- 16-24-ounce lamb shoulder steak, trimmed and cubed into 1½-inch size
- Fresh mint leaves coming from a bunch
- Ground cinnamon, to taste

DIRECTIONS:

1) In a blender, add about one half of pineapple, ginger, garlic, and salt and pulse till smooth.
2) Transfer the mixture into a large bowl.
3) Add chops and coat generously with the mixture.

4) Refrigerate to marinate for about 1-2 hours.
5) Preheat the grill to medium heat. Grease the grill grate.
6) Thread lam, remaining pineapple and mint leaves onto pre-soaked wooden skewers.
7) Grill the kebabs approximately 10 minutes, turning occasionally.
8) Serve when done.

NUTRITION (Per Serving): Calories: 482; Fat: 16g; Phosphorus: 36mg; Potassium: 194mg; Sodium: 31mg; Carbohydrates: 22g; Fiber: 5g; Protein: 377g.

Vegetable

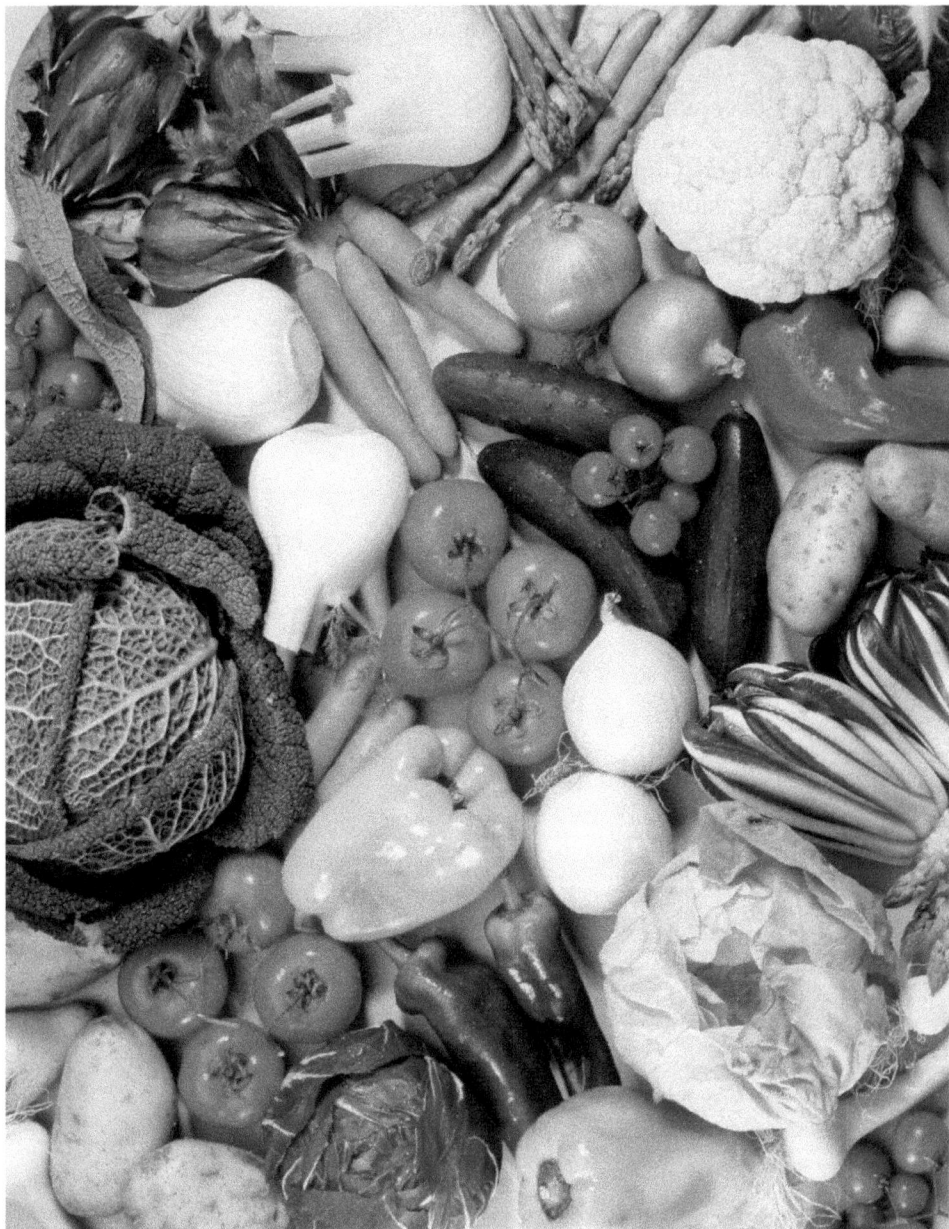

Fried onion rings

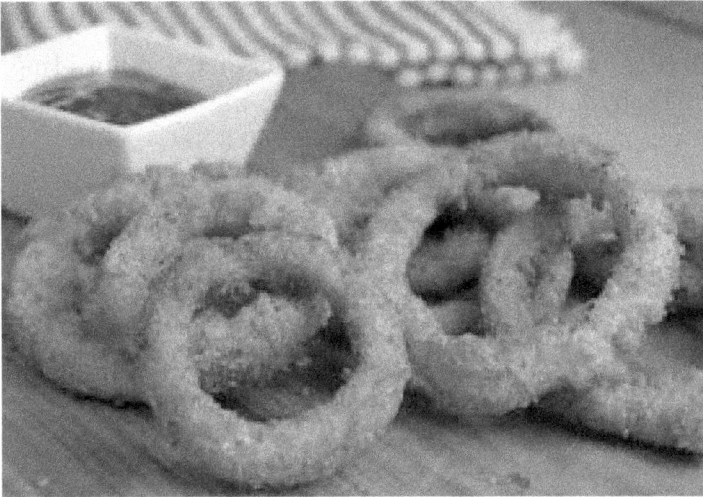

Preparation Time: 10 minutes

Cooking Time: 4-6 minutes

Serving: 1

INGREDIENTS:

- Plain cup plain cornmeal
- ¼ cup all-purpose flour
- 1 teaspoon sugar
- 4 medium onions
- 1 egg, beaten
- ¼ cup water
- ½ cup vegetable oil for frying

DIRECTIONS:

1) Mix cornmeal, flour, and sugar together; set aside.
2) Peel onions and cut crosswise about ¼" thick. Separate into rings.
3) Mix beaten egg and water.
4) Dip rings in egg wash, then into cornmeal mixture.

5) Fry rings for 3-5 minutes in hot vegetable oil, until it turns brown.
6) Drain on a paper towel. Serve hot.

NUTRITION (Per Serving): 162 calories; 0 trans-fat; sodium 11mg; protein 2g; carbohydrate 14g; potassium 99 mg; total fat 11g; cholesterol 27 mg; phosphorus 39 mg; saturated fat1g; fiber 2g; calcium11 mg.

Mediterranean Veggie Pita Sandwich

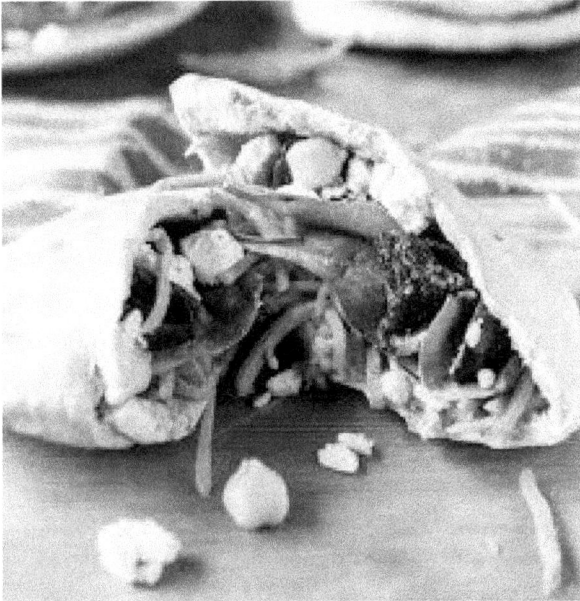

Preparation Time: 10 minutes

Cooking Time: 4-6 minutes

Serving: 1

INGREDIENTS:

- o 1/4 cup chopped carrots
- o A handful of baby spinach
- o 1/4 cup chickpeas
- o 1 teaspoon of crumbled feta cheese
- o 2 teaspoon of fine chopped sun-dried tomatoes
- o 2 teaspoons of chopped kalamata olives
- o Season with salt and pepper

DIRECTIONS:

1) Mix together the chopped carrots, baby spinach, chickpeas, crumbled feta cheese, chopped sun-dried tomatoes, chopped kalamata olives, salt, and pepper.
2) Spread the bath in every pita pant. Sort the rest of the ingredients between the boxes.
3) Eat immediately or pack in a container for lunch.
4) Cool the device if you prepare it for more than 4 hours before eating.

NUTRITION (Per Serving): Calories 287.6; Sodium 716.0 mg; Potassium 263.6 mg; Total Carbohydrate 45.7 g; Dietary Fiber 6.8 g.

Stir-Fried Kale

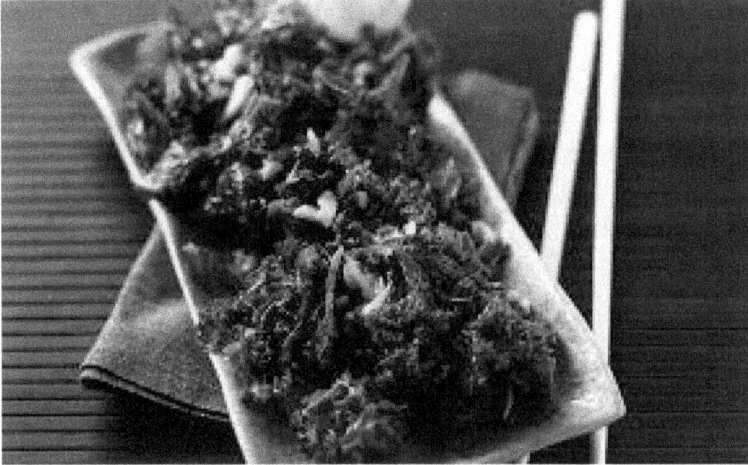

Preparation Time: 10 minutes

Cooking Time: 10 minutes

Serving: 1

INGREDIENTS:

- o   1 tablespoon coconut oil
- o   2 cloves of garlic, minced
- o   1 onion, chopped
- o   2 teaspoons crushed red pepper flakes
- o   4 cups kale, chopped
- o   2 tablespoon water
- o   Salt and pepper to taste

DIRECTIONS:

1) Place a nonstick saucepan on high fire and heat pan for a minute.
2) Add oil and heat for 2 minutes.
3) Stir in garlic and sauté for a minute. Add onions and stir fry for another minute.

4) Add remaining ingredients and stir fry until soft and tender, around 4 minutes.
5) Turn off the fire, let veggies rest while the pan is covered for 3 minutes.
6) Serve and enjoy.

NUTRITION (Per Serving): Calories 37; Total Fat 2g; Saturated Fat 2g; Total Carbs 4g; Net Carbs 3g; Protein 1g; Sugar: 1g; Fiber 1g; Sodium 6mg; Potassium 111mg.

Stir-Fried Bok Choy

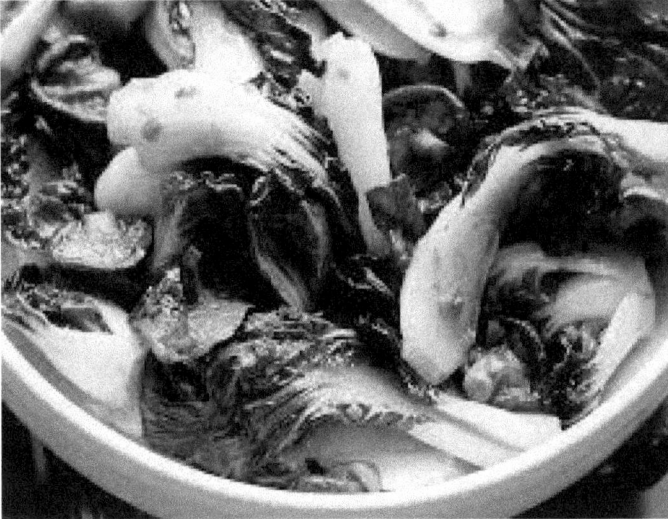

Preparation Time: 10 minutes

Cooking Time: 12 minutes

Serving: 1

INGREDIENTS:

- o 1 tablespoon coconut oil
- o 4 cloves of garlic, minced
- o 1 onion, chopped
- o 2 heads book choy, rinsed and chopped
- o ¼ teaspoon salt
- o ½ teaspoon pepper or more to taste
- o 1 tablespoon sesame seed

DIRECTIONS:

1) Place a nonstick saucepan on high fire and heat pan for a minute.
2) Add sesame seeds and toast for a minute. Transfer to a bowl.
3) In the same pan, add oil and heat for 2 minutes.

4) Stir in garlic and sauté for a minute. Add onions and stir fry for another minute.
5) Add remaining ingredients and stir fry until soft and tender, for around 4 minutes.
6) Turn off the fire, let veggies rest while the pan is covered for 3 minutes.
7) Serve and enjoy.

NUTRITION (Per Serving): Calories 334; Total Fat 20g; Saturated Fat 5g; Total Carbs 36g; Net Carbs 22g; Protein 12g; Sugar: 6g; Fiber 14g; Sodium 731mg; Potassium 1043mg.

Vegetable Curry

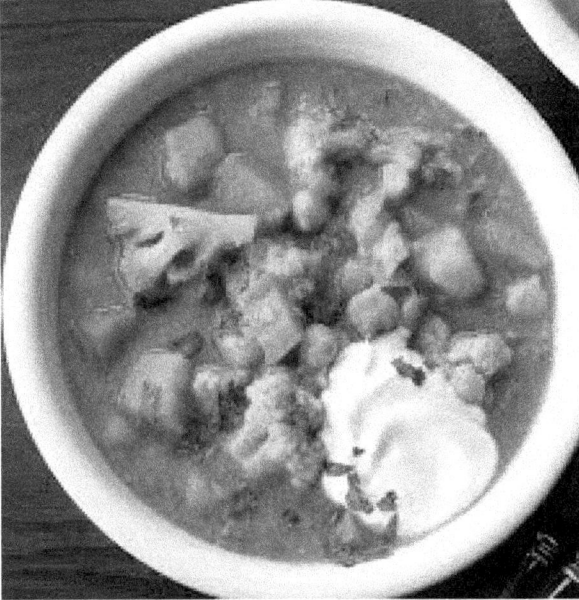

Preparation Time: 10 minutes

Cooking Time: 20 minutes

Serving: 1

INGREDIENTS:

- o 1 tablespoon coconut oil
- o 1 medium onion, chopped
- o 1 teaspoon minced garlic
- o 1 teaspoon minced ginger
- o 2 cup broccoli florets
- o 2 cups fresh spinach leaves
- o 1 tablespoon garam masala
- o ½ cup coconut milk
- o ½ teaspoon salt
- o ½ teaspoon pepper

DIRECTIONS:

8) Place a nonstick pot on high fire and heat it for a minute.
9) Add oil and heat for 2 minutes.
10) Stir in garlic and ginger, sauté for a minute. Add onions and garam masala and stir fry for another minute.
11) Add remaining ingredients, except for spinach leaves, and simmer for 10 minutes.
12) Stir in spinach leaves, turn off the fire, let veggies rest while the pot is covered for 5 minutes.
13) Serve and enjoy.

NUTRITION (Per Serving): Calories 121; Total Fat 11g; Saturated Fat 4g; Total Carbs 6g; Net Carbs 4g; Protein 2g; Sugar: 3g; Fiber 2g; Sodium 315mg; Potassium 266mg

Braised Carrots 'n Kale

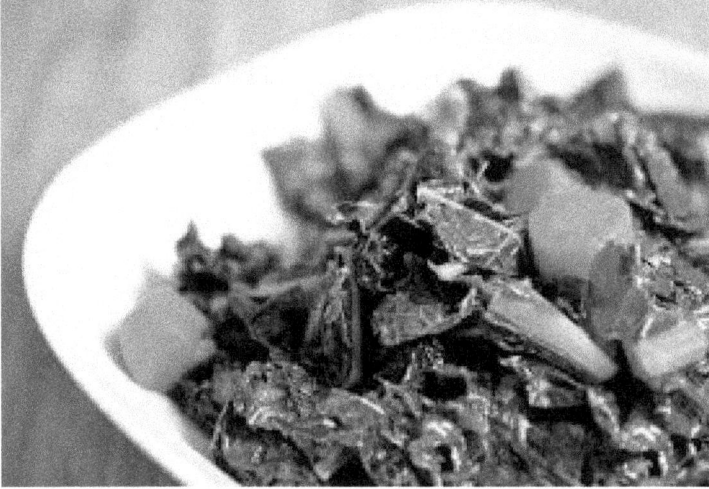

Preparation Time: 10 minutes

Cooking Time: 10 minutes

Serving: 2

INGREDIENTS:

- o   1 tablespoon coconut oil
- o   1 onion, sliced thinly
- o   5 cloves of garlic, minced
- o   3 medium carrots, sliced thinly
- o   10 ounces of kale, chopped
- o   ½ cup water
- o   Salt and pepper to taste
- o   A dash of red pepper flakes

DIRECTIONS:

1) Heat oil in a skillet over medium flame and sauté the onion and garlic until fragrant.
2) Toss in the carrots and stir for 1 minute. Add the kale and water. Season with salt and pepper to taste.

3) Close the lid and allow to simmer for 5 minutes.
4) Sprinkle with red pepper flakes.
5) Serve and enjoy.

NUTRITION (Per Serving): Calories 161; Total Fat 8g; Saturated Fat 1g; Total Carbs 20g; Net Carbs 14g; Protein 8g; Sugar: 6g; Fiber 6g; Sodium 63mg; Potassium 900mg

Butternut Squash Hummus

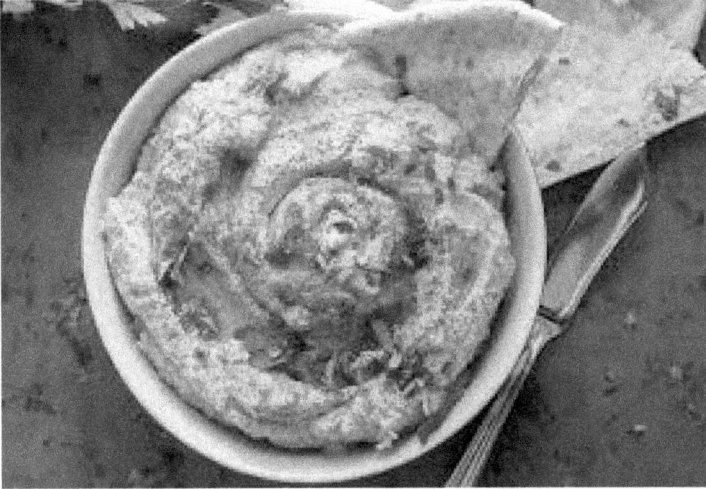

Preparation Time: 10 minutes

Cooking Time: 15 minutes

Serving: 1

INGREDIENTS:

- o 2 pounds butternut squash, seeded and peeled
- o 1 tablespoon olive oil
- o ¼ cup tahini
- o 2 tablespoons lemon juice
- o 2 cloves of garlic, minced
- o Salt and pepper to taste

DIRECTIONS:

1) Heat the oven to 300^0F.
2) Coat the butternut squash with olive oil.
3) Place in a baking dish and bake for 15 minutes in the oven.
4) Once the squash is cooked, place in a food processor together with the rest of the ingredients.
5) Pulse until smooth.

6) Place in individual containers.
7) Put a label and store it in the fridge.
8) Allow warming at room temperature before heating in the microwave oven.
9) Serve with carrots or celery sticks.

NUTRITION (Per Serving): Calories 109; Total Fat 6g; Saturated Fat 0.8g; Total Carbs 15g; Net Carbs 11g; Protein 2g; Sugar: 3g; Fiber 4g; Sodium 14mg; Potassium 379mg.

Stir-Fried Gingery Veggies

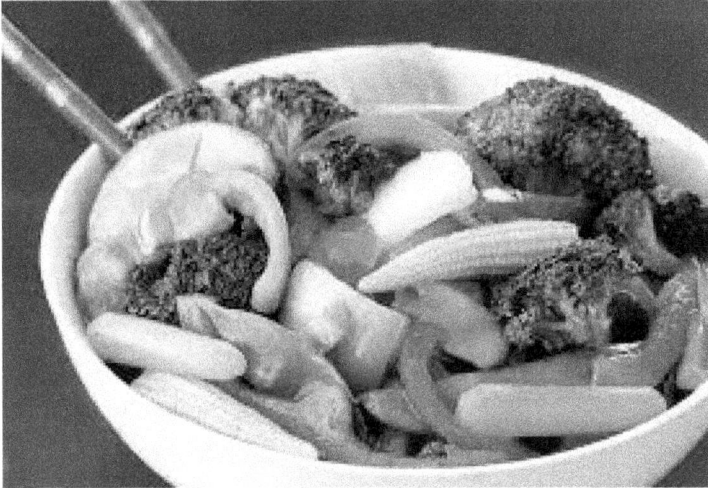

Preparation Time: 10 minutes

Cooking Time: 10 minutes

Serving: 1

INGREDIENTS:

- 1 tablespoon oil
- 3 cloves of garlic, minced
- 1 onion, chopped
- 1 thumb-size ginger, sliced
- 1 tablespoon water
- 1 large carrot, peeled and julienned
- 1 large green bell pepper, seeded and julienned
- 1 large yellow bell pepper, seeded and julienned
- 1 large red bell pepper, seeded and julienned
- 1 zucchini, julienned
- Salt and pepper to taste

DIRECTIONS:

1) Heat oil in a nonstick saucepan over a high flame and sauté the garlic, onion, and ginger until fragrant.
2) Stir in the rest of the ingredients.
3) Keep on stirring for at least 5 minutes until vegetables are tender.
4) Serve and enjoy.

NUTRITION (Per Serving): Calories 70; Total Fat 4g; Saturated Fat 1g; Total Carbs 9g; Net Carbs 7g; Protein 1g; Sugar: 4g; Fiber 2g; Sodium 273mg; Potassium 263mg

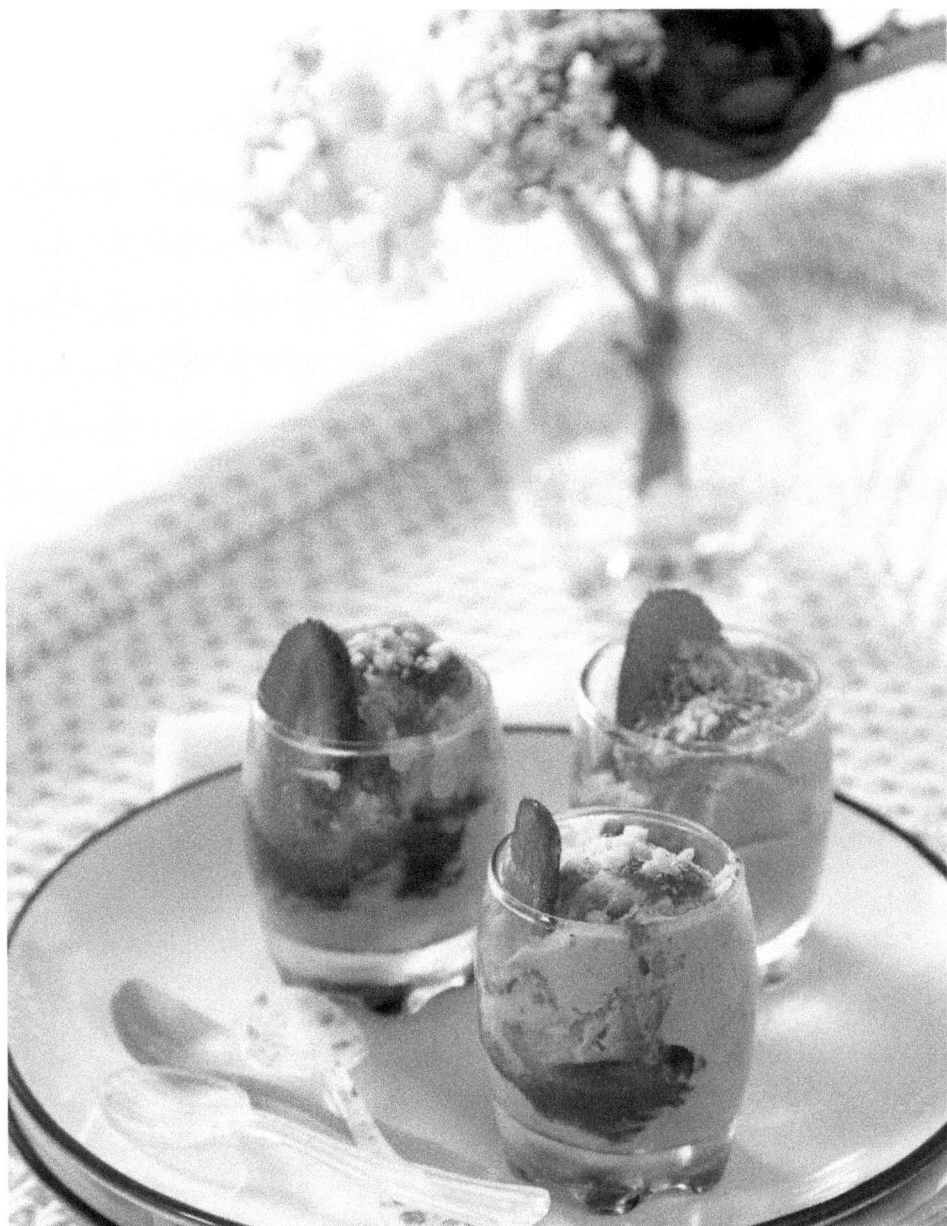

Dessert

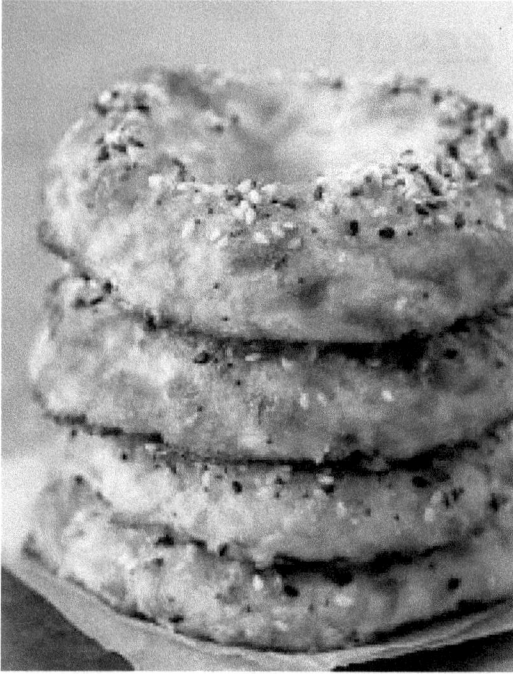

Cauliflower Bagel

Preparation Time: 10 minutes

Cooking Time: 30 minutes

Serving: 1

INGREDIENTS:

- 1 large cauliflower; divided into florets and roughly chopped
- ¼ cup nutritional yeast
- ¼ cup almond flour
- ½ teaspoon garlic powder
- 1 ½ teaspoon fine sea salt
- 2 whole eggs
- 1 tablespoon sesame seeds

DIRECTIONS:

1) Preheat your oven to 400 °F
2) Line a baking sheet with parchment paper, keep it on the side.
3) Blend cauliflower in a food processor and transfer to a bowl.
4) Add nutritional yeast, almond flour, garlic powder, and salt to a bowl and mix.
5) Take another bowl and whisk in eggs, add to cauliflower mix.
6) Give the dough a stir.
7) Incorporate the mix into the egg mix.

8) Make balls from the dough, making a hole using your thumb into each ball.
9) Arrange them on your prepped sheet, flattening them into bagel shapes.
10) Sprinkle sesame seeds and bake for half an hour.
11) Remove the oven and let them cool, enjoy!

NUTRITION (Per Serving): Calories: 152; Fat: 10g; Phosphorus: 20mg; Potassium: 194mg; Sodium: 30mg; Carbohydrates: 4g; Protein: 4g.

Vanilla Biscuits

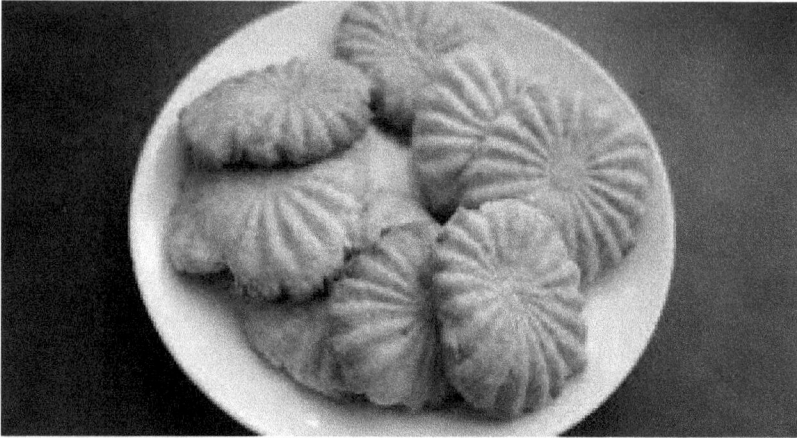

Preparation Time: 15 minutes

Cooking Time: 40 minutes

Serving: 1

INGREDIENTS:

- 5 eggs
- ½ cup coconut flour
- ½ cup wheat flour
- 1/3 cup Erythritol
- 1 teaspoon vanilla extract
- Cooking spray

DIRECTIONS:

1) Crack the eggs in the mixing bowl and mix it up with the help of the hand mixer.
2) Then add Erythritol and keep mixing the egg mixture until it will be changed into the lemon color.
3) Then add wheat flour, coconut flour, and vanilla extract.
4) Mix it for 30 seconds.
5) Spray the baking tray with cooking spray.
6) Pour the biscuit mixture in the tray and flatten it.

7) Bake it for 40 minutes at 350^0 F.
8) When the biscuit is cooked, cut it into squares and serve.

NUTRITION (Per Serving): Calories 132; Fat 4.7; Fiber 4.3; Phosphorus: 21mg; Potassium: 145mg; Sodium: 20mg; Carbs 28.3; Protein 7

Semolina Pudding

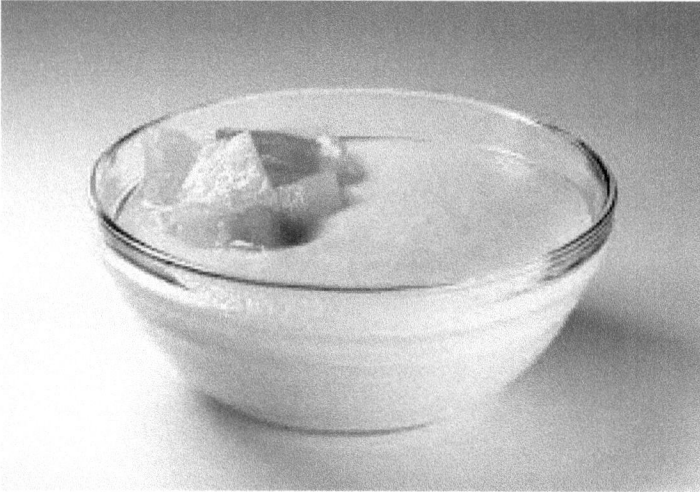

Preparation Time: 15 minutes

Cooking Time: 7 minutes

Serving: 1

INGREDIENTS:

- ½ cup organic almond milk
- ½ cup milk
- 1/3 cup semolina
- 1 tablespoon butter
- ¼ teaspoon cornstarch
- ½ teaspoon almond extract

DIRECTIONS:

1) Pour almond milk and milk in the saucepan.
2) Bring it to boil and add semolina and cornstarch.
3) Mix the ingredients until homogenous and simmer them for 1 minute.
4) After this, add almond extract and butter. Stir well and close the lid.

5) Remove the pudding from the heat and leave for 10 minutes.
6) Then mix it again and transfer in the serving ramekins.

NUTRITION (Per Serving): calories 201; fat 7.9; fiber 1.1; Phosphorus: 30mg; Potassium: 74mg; Sodium: 26mg; carbs 25.7; protein 5.8.

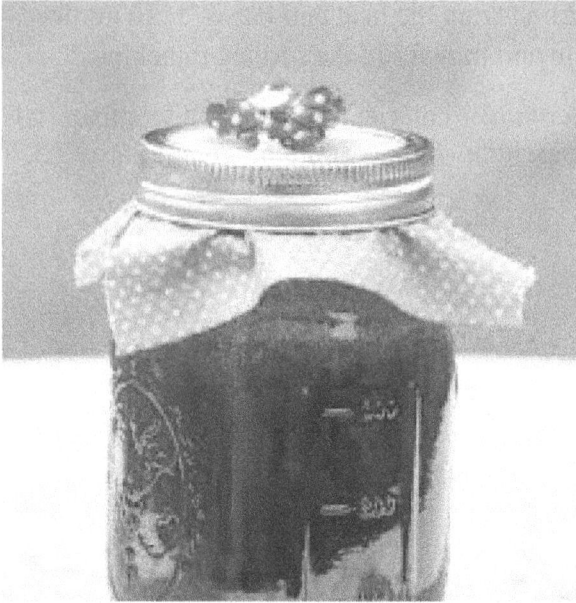

Watermelon Jelly

Preparation Time: 30 minutes

Cooking Time: 5 minutes

Serving: 2

INGREDIENTS:

- 8 oz watermelon
- 1 tablespoon gelatin powder

DIRECTIONS:

1) Make the juice from the watermelon with the help of the fruit juicer.
2) Combine 5 tablespoons of watermelon juice and 1 tablespoon of gelatin powder. Stir it and leave for 5 minutes.
3) Then heat the remaining watermelon juice until warm, add gelatin mixture, and heat it over the medium heat until gelatin is dissolved.
4) Then remove the liquid from the heat and put it in the silicone molds.
5) Freeze the jelly for 30 minutes in the freezer or 4 hours in the fridge.

NUTRITION (Per Serving): Calories 46; Fat 0.2; Fiber 0.4; Phosphorus: 10mg; Potassium: 200mg; Sodium: 12mg; Carbs 8.5; Protein 3.7.

Greek Cookies

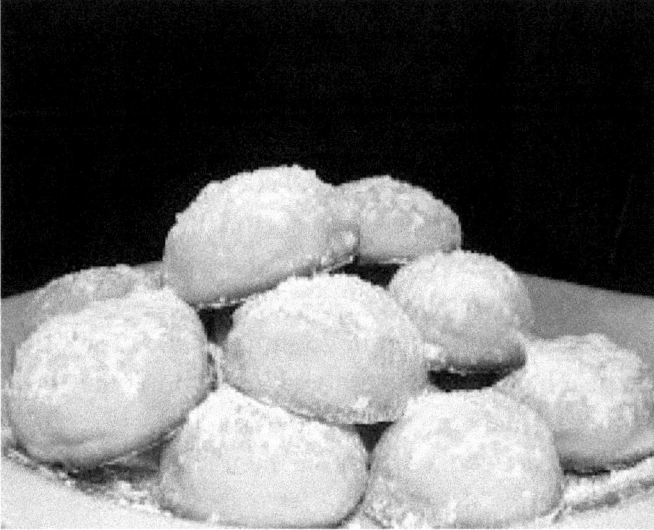

Preparation Time: 20 minutes

Cooking Time: 25 minutes

Serving: 1

INGREDIENTS:

- ½ cup plain yogurt
- ½ teaspoon baking powder
- 2 tablespoons Erythritol
- 1 teaspoon almond extract
- ½ teaspoon ground clove
- ½ teaspoon orange zest; grated
- 3 tablespoons walnuts; chopped
- 1 cup wheat flour
- 1 teaspoon butter, softened
- 1 tablespoon honey
- 3 tablespoons water

DIRECTIONS:

1) In the mixing bowl mix up together Plain yogurt, baking powder, Erythritol, almond extract, ground cloves orange zest, flour, and butter.
2) Knead the non-sticky dough. Add olive oil if the dough is very sticky and knead it well.
3) Then make the log from the dough and cut it into small pieces.
4) Roll every piece of dough into the balls and transfer in the baking paper-lined baking tray.
5) Press the balls gently and bake for 25 minutes at 350^0 F.
6) Meanwhile, heat honey and water together. Simmer the liquid for 1 minute and remove from the heat.
7) When the cookies are cooked, remove them from the oven and let them cool for 5 minutes.
8) Then pour the cookies with sweet honey water and sprinkle with walnuts.
9) Let the cookies cool, before serving.

NUTRITION (Per Serving): Calories 134; Fat 3.4; Fiber 0.9; Phosphorus: 17mg; Potassium: 100mg; Sodium: 18mg; Carbs 26.1; Protein 4.3

Baked Figs with Honey

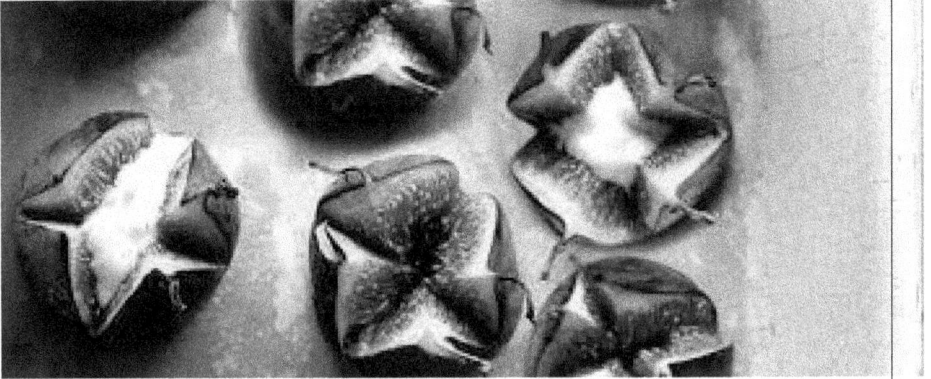

Preparation Time: 10 minutes

Cooking Time: 15 minutes

Serving: 1

INGREDIENTS:

- 4 figs
- 4 teaspoons honey
- 1 oz blue cheese, chopped

DIRECTIONS:

1) Make the cross cuts in the figs and fill them with chopped blue cheese.
2) Then sprinkle the figs with honey and wrap in the foil.
3) Bake the figs for 15 minutes at 355^0 F.
4) Remove the figs from the foil and transfer it in the serving plates.

NUTRITION (Per Serving): Calories 94; Fat 2.2; Fiber 1.9; Phosphorus: 19mg; Potassium: 50mg; Sodium: 31mg; Carbs 18.1; Protein 2.2.

Cream Strawberry Pies

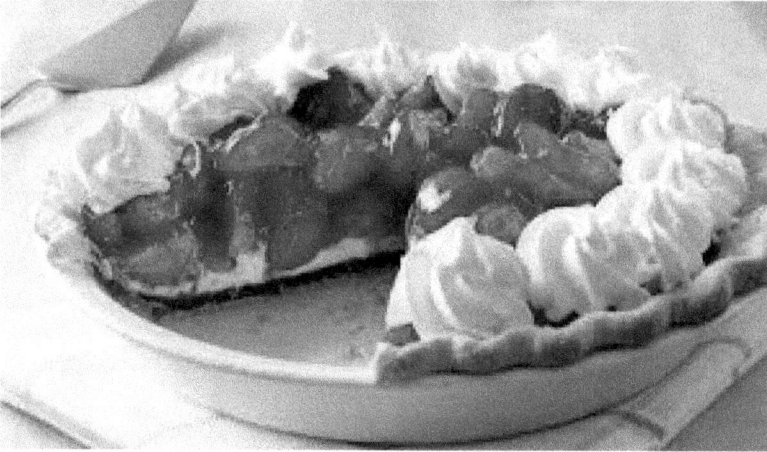

Preparation Time: 20 minutes

Cooking Time: 15 minutes

Serving: 1

INGREDIENTS:

- o 1 cup strawberries
- o 7 oz puff pastry
- o 3 teaspoons butter, softened
- o 3 teaspoons Erythritol
- o ¼ teaspoon ground nutmeg
- o 4 teaspoons cream

DIRECTIONS:

1) Roll up the puff pastry and cut it into 6 squares.
2) Slice the strawberries.
3) Grease every puff pastry square with butter and then place the sliced strawberries on it.
4) Sprinkle the strawberry square with cream, ground nutmeg, and Erythritol.

5) Secure the edges of the puff pastry square in the shape of a pie.
6) Line the baking tray with baking paper.
7) Transfer the pies in the tray and place the tray in the oven.
8) Bake the pies for 15 minutes at 375^0 F.

NUTRITION (Per Serving): Calories 209; Fat 14.8; Phosphorus: 30mg; Potassium: 124mg; Sodium: 29mg; Fiber 1; Carbs 19.4; Protein 2.6.

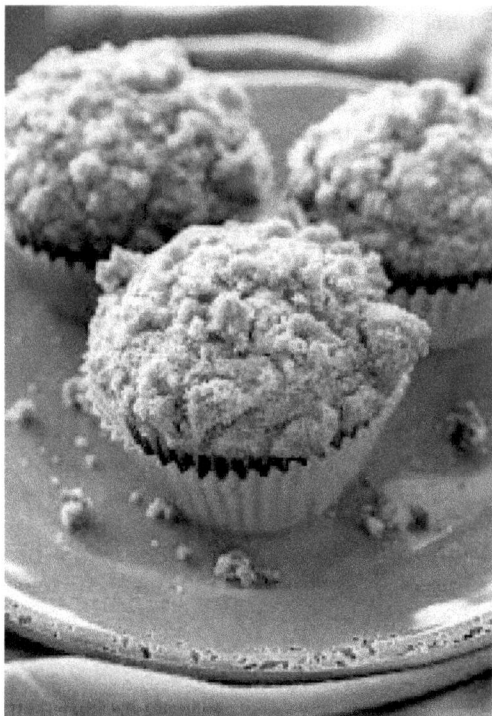

Banana Muffins

Preparation Time: 10 minutes

Cooking Time: 12 minutes

Serving: 1

INGREDIENTS:

o   4 tablespoons wheat flour
o   2 bananas, peeled
o   1 tablespoon plain yogurt
o   ½ teaspoon baking powder
o   ¼ teaspoon lemon juice
o   1 teaspoon vanilla extract

DIRECTIONS:

1) Mash the bananas with the help of the fork.
2) Then combine mashed bananas with flour, yogurt, baking powder, and lemon juice.
3) Add vanilla extract and stir the batter until smooth.
4) Fill ½ part of every muffin mold with banana batter and bake them for 12 minutes at 365^0 F.
5) Chill the muffins and remove them from the muffin molds.

NUTRITION (Per Serving): calories 87; fat 0.3; Phosphorus: 36mg; Potassium: 194mg; Sodium: 31mg; fiber 1.8; carbs 20.2; protein 1.7.

Measurement Conversion Chart

American and British Variances					
Term	**Abbrevia tion**	**Nationa lity**	**Dry or liquid**	**Metric equivalent**	**Equivalent in context**
cup	c., C.		usually liquid	237 milliliters	16 tablespoons or 8 ounces
ounce	fl oz, fl. oz.	America n	liquid only	29.57 milliliters	
		British	either	28.41 milliliters	
gallon	gal.	America n	liquid only	3.785 liters	4 quarts
		British	either	4.546 liters	4 quarts
inch	in, in.			2.54 centimeters	
ounce	oz, oz.	America n	dry	28.35 grams	1/16 pound
			liquid	see OUNCE	see OUNCE
pint	p., pt.	America n	liquid	0.473 liter	1/8 gallon or 16 ounces
			dry	0.551 liter	1/2 quart
		British	either	0.568 liter	
pound	lb.		dry	453.592 grams	16 ounces
Quart	q., qt, qt.	America n	liquid	0.946 liter	1/4 gallon or 32 ounces
			dry	1.101 liters	2 pints
		British	either	1.136 liters	
Teaspoo n	t., tsp., tsp		either	about 5 milliliters	1/3 tablespoon
Tablesp oon	T., tbs., tbsp.		either	about 15 milliliters	3 teaspoons or 1/2 ounce

Volume (Liquid)

American Standard (Cups & Quarts)	American Standard (Ounces)	Metric (Milliliters & Liters)
2 tbsp.	1 fl. oz.	30 ml
1/4 cup	2 fl. oz.	60 ml
1/2 cup	4 fl. oz.	125 ml
1 cup	8 fl. oz.	250 ml
1 1/2 cups	12 fl. oz.	375 ml
2 cups or 1 pint	16 fl. oz.	500 ml
4 cups or 1 quart	32 fl. oz.	1000 ml or 1 liter
1 gallon	128 fl. oz.	4 liters

Volume (Dry)

American Standard	Metric
1/8 teaspoon	5 ml
1/4 teaspoon	1 ml
1/2 teaspoon	2 ml
3/4 teaspoon	4 ml
1 teaspoon	5 ml
1 tablespoon	15 ml
1/4 cup	59 ml
1/3 cup	79 ml
1/2 cup	118 ml
2/3 cup	158 ml
3/4 cup	177 ml
1 cup	225 ml
2 cups or 1 pint	450 ml
3 cups	675 ml
4 cups or 1 quart	1 liter
1/2 gallon	2 liters
1 gallon	4 liters

Dry Measure Equivalents

3 teaspoons	1 tablespoon	1/2 ounce	14.3 grams
2 tablespoons	1/8 cup	1 ounce	28.3 grams
4 tablespoons	1/4 cup	2 ounces	56.7 grams
5 1/3 tablespoons	1/3 cup	2.6 ounces	75.6 grams
8 tablespoons	1/2 cup	4 ounces	113.4 grams
12 tablespoons	3/4 cup	6 ounces	.375 pound
32 tablespoons	2 cups	16 ounces	1 pound

Oven Temperatures

American Standard	Metric
250° F	130° C
300° F	150° C
350° F	180° C
400° F	200° C
450° F	230° C

Weight (Mass)

American Standard (Ounces)	Metric (Grams)
1/2 ounce	15 grams
1 ounce	30 grams
3 ounces	85 grams
3.75 ounces	100 grams
4 ounces	115 grams
8 ounces	225 grams
12 ounces	340 grams
16 ounces or 1 pound	450 grams